# PRAISE FOR

## HOME MASSAGE
*Transforming Family Life Through the Healing Power of Touch*

"This book is well-crafted, practical, creative, innovative and accessible. Highly recommended for all those who value the role of touch and intimacy in their lives."
—Mariana Caplan, Ph.D. , author of *To Touch is to Live*

---

"The healing power of massage therapy must be promoted in all appropriate venues—and healthy touch in the home is a vital component of creating harmony and happiness. From infants to seniors, we all need touch, and *Home Massage*, by Chuck Fata and Suzette Hodnett, with its focus on relationship, stress relief, body image and nonsexual touch, provides an important stepping stone on the path to peace in our world."
—Joseph D. Doyle, president and CEO, The Doyle Group, publisher of MASSAGE Magazine and Chiropractic Economics magazine

---

"This book does it all! Simple yet profound, great for beginners or professionals, filled with insight and wisdom. Chuck had the best hands of any bodyworker I have ever known and the compassion and love he could express through his touch was truly astonishing."
—Dr. Vincent Medici D.C. and Ph.D., Biochemistry, Curriculum Director for Western Sciences at The Shiatsu Massage School of CA

---

"This book offers insight into touch that many massage text books do not offer. It is the conversation about how touch communicates, the discussions of honor, respect and presence, and the methods of being comfortable in one's own body and mind, that are not always available, but are extremely important to introduce to the student of touch and future therapists. I would recommend using this book as a classroom text for both the casual student and the professional one."
—Tania Clutter, LMT, Instructor, Everest College

---

"Those of us who know and live healthy touch can't even imagine ourselves without it. This is a book that is long overdue. When one opens his heart to healthy touch, the possibilities are unlimited."
—Michael Young, NCTMB, Founder of RUIT (Repetitive Use Injury Therapy)

"This beautiful, comprehensive guide to massage is a gift for our families and loved ones, in teaching each of us how to support one another though the healing power of touch. The heartfelt photos tell the story so eloquently of creating quality connection, being present and giving to those in our lives who give so much to us each and everyday. And there is nothing more profound than cultivating the skills for massage in our children and an appreciation of the power it has to bring us together in harmony and to help us heal both physically and emotionally. This book is a gem to be shared with friends and family and generations of a lifetime."
    —Tara Grodjesk, President and Founder, Tara Spa Therapy
    Certified Holistic Health Educator, Massage Therapist, Ayurvedic Practitioner

"Chuck and Suzette have succeeded in creating a fun, easy-to-follow guide to home massage. The book covers everything from creating a safe environment to a full massage routine with basic strokes. Written for beginners, it's guaranteed to enhance your family life as you discover the joy and happiness of healing touch."
    —Tomas Nani, Founder, Earthlite Massage Tables

"What can be as simple, and as wonderful, as a touch? This book explores this concept in clear, concise language and pictures so that ANYONE can partake of one of the greatest gifts of being human. As a public librarian I am often wary of massage books and whether the message within will be appropriate to my patrons. Thankfully, with books such as this, the gift of touch can be explored in a safe and nurturing environment. When we get a copy in our collection I plan on checking it out many times!"
    —Terry Oxley, Librarian II, Youth Services, Velma Teague Branch

"As a retired educator and former superintendent, I know the importance of social interaction and the role human touch plays in the development of children both in and out of the classroom. In these days when we are sensitive to and limit 'touch' in schools, we can't lose site of this aspect of being human. There is much stress in the modern school environment and plenty of studies about the positive effects of massage on decreasing stress. In *Home Massage* by Chuck Fata and Suzette Hodnett, there are clear ways to have parents and their children together learn to experience the positive effect of touch which can better prepare them to meet the demands of school, both academic and social. This book is an important tool to provide improved health for all who utilize the steps it provides."
    —Dr. Laura McGaughey, retired educator and former superintendent

"This book is just lovely and well written. The authors did a wonderful job in covering the topic of massage for everyone and demonstrating how easy it is to put the power of touch in every household. Children to grandparents will love this book."
> —Lynda Solien-Wolfe LMT, NCTMB, Vice-Chair of the Florida Board of Massage Therapy, President of the Solwolfe Resource Group, Inc.

---

"I've been getting massage regularly for 25 years and wish my family had started 25 years before that. I'm the 'Massage Dad' in our house and thankful for the opportunity to give to my family. This book is a must have and every family will benefit from its common sense approach to family healing."
> —Allan Share, President, Day Spa Association, International Medical Spa Association

---

"Chuck and Suzette break new ground with an excellent book designed to bring the healing benefits of touch through massage into our daily life. They are a clear voice on how respect, honor, and appropriate touch learned on the massage table can return intimacy and loving touch to family life. Every family should have this book to use and peruse daily."
> —Bruce Eatchel, GM and VP, Stronglite Massage Tables

---

"Touch is vital to the health of body, mind and soul. Yet, because of the transgressions of a few, many Western societies are legislating against touch in public institutions. This is not the answer. The solution is to teach people how to touch in a nurturing and safe way. *Home Massage* does this beautifully within the family setting. All members of the family are included—young and old, healthy and ill, male and female, parent and child, brother and sister. Bravo!"
> —Gayle MacDonald, *Medicine Hands: Massage Therapy for People with Cancer*

---

The wonderful principles and techniques described in this book reveal the real healing power of touch, which is often neglected in families but can make such a difference in our physical, emotional and mental health.
> —Dr. Chris Elisabeth Gilbert, M.D., Ph.D., author of *Dr. Chris's A, B, C's of Health* and *The French Stethoscope*

We recommend you also consult the companion DVD to this book:

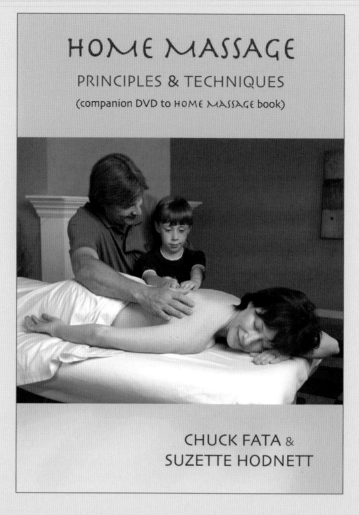

HOME MASSAGE
PRINCIPLES & TECHNIQUES
(companion DVD to HOME MASSAGE book)

CHUCK FATA &
SUZETTE HODNETT

With step-by-step instructions from certified wellness experts, this DVD demonstrates how anyone can use massage to bring health and connection back into family life. Designed for the nonprofessional, the 47-minute disc is divided into three sections. Section one discusses the philosophy and important principles of home massage. Then, section two offers easy-to-follow directions showing all aspects of giving an effective full-body massage. Finally, section three presents ideas for bringing home massage into daily life with children, adolescents, the elderly, spouses, and infants. This invaluable resource will allow viewers to discover the healing benefits of touch in their own home with the people they know and trust.

*Available from:*

• your local bookstore

• the author's website:
www.tchcomemassage.com

• the publisher's website:
www.findhornpress.com

# HOME MASSAGE

## Transforming Family Life
## Through the Healing Power of Touch

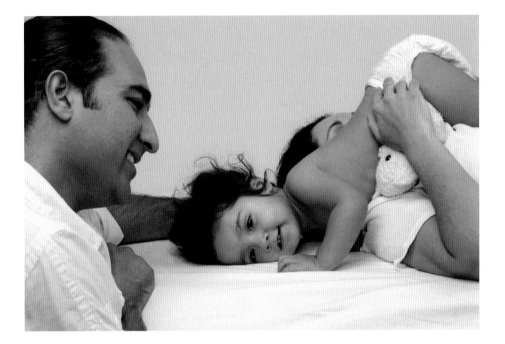

# CHUCK FATA &
# SUZETTE HODNETT

MASSAGE CONSULTANT
JACKIE SLOAN

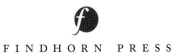

FINDHORN PRESS

First published by Findhorn Press 2011

ISBN 978-1-84409-559-9

British Library Cataloguing-in-Publication Data.
A catalogue record for this book is available from the British Library.

Printed and bound in China

1 2 3 4 5 6 7 8 9 10 17 16 15 14 13 12 13 12 11

Published by
Findhorn Press
117-121 High Street
Forres IV36 1AB
Scotland, UK

t +44(0)1309 690582
f +44(0)131 777 2711
e info@findhornpress.com
www.findhornpress.com

In loving memory of

**Chuck Fata**
whose healing hands and heart touched us all

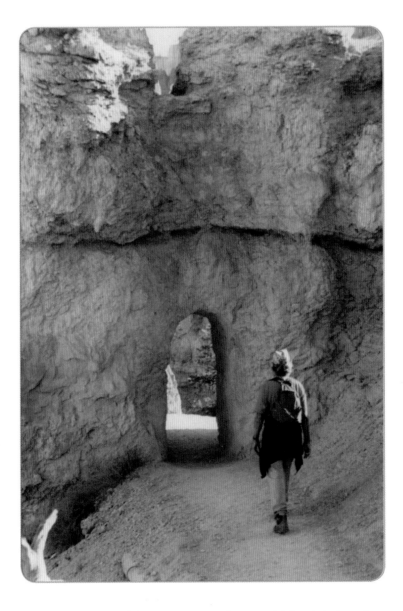

His vision and journey continue within this book.

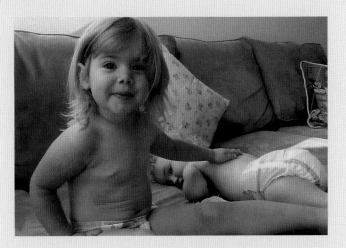

Touch is our first language.

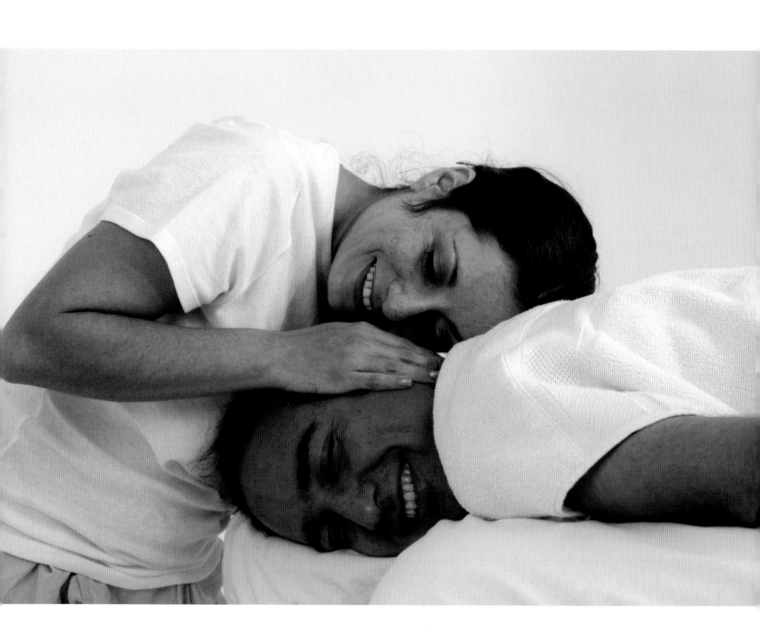

The best environment to provide healing touch
is in the safety of our home and the "toucher" would be
a husband, wife, other family member or trusted friend.

—Mariana Caplan, Ph.D, *To Touch is To Live*

# CONTENTS

## Introduction

## Section One — Understanding Home Massage

## Section Two — Learning Home Massage

## Section Three — Bringing Home Massage Into Your Life

## Conclusion

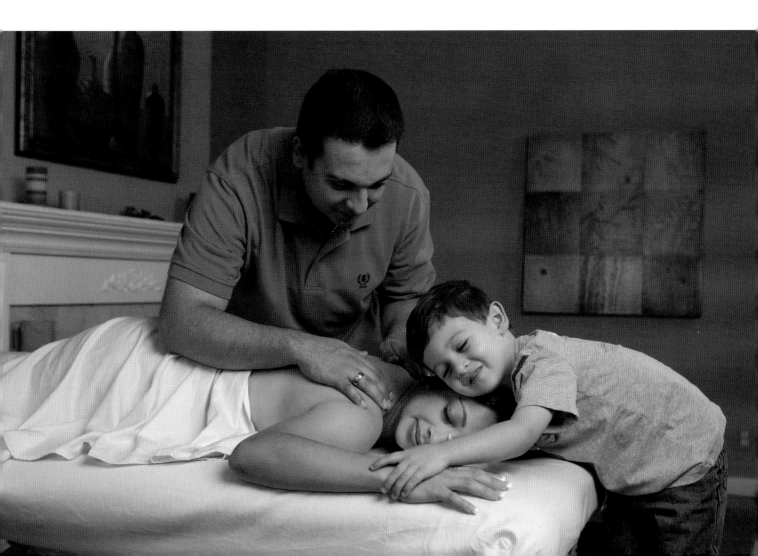

# FOREWORD

If you are holding this book in your hands, you have already made a conscious step closer to connecting with your loved ones. Your innate senses are reminding you of how good it feels to be touched or to touch someone. Those same senses "know" that touch relaxes, heals, connects, and communicates. It can be as simple as a warm feeling of security and acceptance or as powerful as to create mental, emotional and physical shifts in our lives. It is the way most of us were touched as children—unabashed, unrestrained, free and unashamed. But when is the last time you remember touching someone or being touched in that way?

Our social upbringing, our poor experiences with touch, our physical and emotional injuries and the rules and regulations imposed on us at our workplaces and schools have slowly and surreptitiously led us to put up barriers so that we might find ourselves not touching or being touched for days. Human touch is as vital to our physical and emotional health as food and water. Would we consider going without food and water?

In 2004, Chuck Fata was asked to teach a 15-hour massage class for the students at the University of California at Irvine. He took the challenge and found that they were starving for touch and yet full of apprehensions. Aware of this, he opted to teach what we knew to be under the surface of healthy, human touch. He taught about respect, honor and nurturing intentions, of being present and aware, of being comfortable with touch and comfortable in one's body. Techniques followed, and with these concepts in place, Chuck and the students created a safe, nurturing, loving environment free from sexual intonations and fears of being hurt. Creativity, trust and relaxation then happened naturally. I came to assist Chuck with this first group and was truly fascinated by what I saw. These students looked like professionals after only four hours. Word spread, and it became the most popular class in the department. Chuck and I continued our research, discussions and teaching. With great fortune we added life coach, Tai Chi sandan and co-author of this book, Suzette Hodnett. With her psychological expertise and her East/West perspectives, together we recognized we had a different approach and the desire to bring it to the general public.

*Home Massage: Transforming Family Life Through the Healing Power of Touch* is one of our gateways to present these concepts to the world around us. Years were spent in its development. We have seen that the introduction to these principles is what makes massage easy to learn and extremely effective. TC Home Massage bridges massage techniques with the art of massage. This is rare, even in the professional world. There is much more to massage than structural change and this book explores the depth of human touch in clear language, simple directions and heartwarming photography.

Our lives are fast-paced and there seems to be no time for rest, peace and introspection. If one could only "take a breath." This book offers us that breath. Our society is hesitant to touch and fears improper touch. This book is an invitation to make proper touch a household word. Our families and friends often miss out on our deepest communication—loving touch. This book shares a path to bring the lessons learned on the massage table into our relationships and our daily lives.

Touch is our innate wisdom. It is not something we need to learn, but something we need to remember. What better place than with our trusted friends and family to return to our natural ability of healing touch through massage?

Turn the pages to learn the principles beneath touch, the techniques for a basic massage and everyday methods to use this gift to bring your family and friends closer. Whether you have five minutes or an evening to spend, every touch shared is a communication. Don't miss the opportunity.

—JACKIE SLOAN, CMT
CO-FOUNDER, TCHM

# A MESSAGE FROM THE AUTHORS

It's a home run and the Yankees have won the World Series.

In that moment, in front of thousands of people with millions of others watching on television, the winning team rushes to the middle of the field and embraces each other with hugs, expressing the joy of victory through the language of touch.

Elsewhere in that very same moment, the father of an 18-year-old exchange student preparing to leave on a flight to a foreign land resists hugging his daughter in public. While a baseball team is hugging in front of millions, a father and daughter are not willing to physically and emotionally connect in public. Observing these extreme attitudes regarding touch has captured my imagination.

We are all comfortable with some kind of touch. For some it is a handshake; for others, a hug. But we all have a "touch threshold" that keeps us from opening further our body, our heart, and our mind to the countless gifts of touch.

During the past ten years, while teaching massage to the general public, I have seen years of touch inhibition disappear as people of all ages become comfortable with touch through giving and receiving massage. I have seen others already comfortable with touch begin sharing massage with their families, making touch a greater part of their daily lives. One of my students contacted me seven years after taking my massage class to tell me how it had changed her life. I would find that hard to believe, but I have heard similar stories from other students. This is the power of clear boundaries and nonsexual touch. It is the power of honoring yourself and honoring others. It is the power of becoming comfortable giving and receiving healing touch. It is the power of touching someone in a reverent way.

When we become comfortable massaging someone for ten minutes or for an hour, we are transformed. The true magic of massage comes from the duration of touch that extends to us the gift of an unlimited potential to heal. Through home massage, we return to the powerful language of touch we knew as a child but have since forgotten as adults. We remember how relaxation feels. We connect with those we love. And we bring touch into our daily lives as a way to communicate with our children, spouses, relatives, and friends.

I invite you to learn the art of Touch Communications Home Massage (TCHM) and discover the healing benefits of touch for yourself.

—CHUCK FATA

As far back as I can remember, "taking turns" was a part of my vocabulary and my life. One of my first memories is of massaging my dad's back. He didn't know about the many benefits of home massage, but he was a teacher who stood in front of his class all day and appreciated a good back massage after school. In return, he would massage me while he watched television. I will never forget the feeling of his single hand enveloping my tiny back. In those moments, I felt safe, loved, and calm.

Although I was raised in an alcoholic family with unpredictable stress and trauma, even a few minutes of massage exchange from a parent or sibling would return me to a feeling of calm. Some nights I would even lie in bed and massage my own arms, putting myself to sleep. My sisters and I would always exchange massage—before bed, on vacation, and when we were bored. In the car, massage was the only thing allowing us to cross the "imaginary line" that separated our places in the back seat.

Life comes full circle and, years later, as both my parents were dying of cancer, I comforted them through massage. It was our conversation without words. It made them feel better and less alone. It made me feel helpful and loving. As they grew weaker, massage turned to gentle touch, then to a held hand in their final moments.

Working in the field of psychotherapy for over twenty years, I have seen what happens when touch invades and damages and what happens when touch embraces and heals. I have listened to painful stories of abusive touch that scarred a child's soul for a lifetime. I have seen how loving touch or a forgiving hug—father to son or husband to wife—can heal a deep hurt that may have taken years in talk therapy. I have seen the lonely and depressed who craved and needed touch, but had no place to either receive or give it. I have seen discomfort with touch passed on from generation to generation.

It has been said that touching is the true revolution. In our Touch Communications Home Massage (TCHM) workshops, I continue to see mother and daughter, father and son, friends and couples reach a place that defies explanation. Quiet. Present. Respectful. Calm. Loving. Touched. A place of freedom, safety, and connection. We need more of this—as individuals, as families, and as a culture.

We have this amazing gift at our fingertips that costs nothing, can go anywhere and makes us feel relaxed, loved, and healthy. I used to joke that my perfect world would be that anywhere, anytime, we could exchange back rubs with our family and friends. I have always wondered why more people weren't "taking turns." Now they can. Welcome to Touch Communications Home Massage—for family and friends.

—SUZETTE HODNETT

# INTRODUCTION

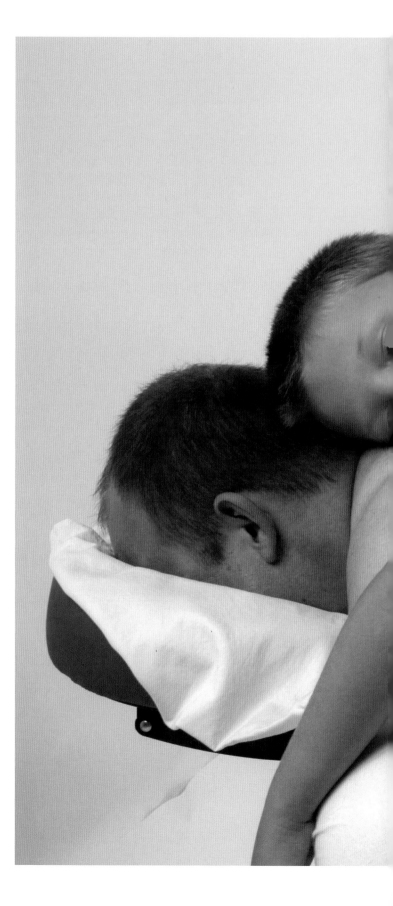

Who says massage has to be only in the hands of the professionals? Anyone can do it! Countless individuals like yourself are beginning to use one of the oldest healing therapies known to man—massage—to bring health and connection back into their daily lives. Someday every home will have a massage table—as natural a piece of furniture as the living room sofa. More and more families are exchanging massage and allowing healing touch to be an integral part of their daily lives. Now you can experience the transformative benefits of bringing massage into your home.

Home massage is an idea whose time has come.

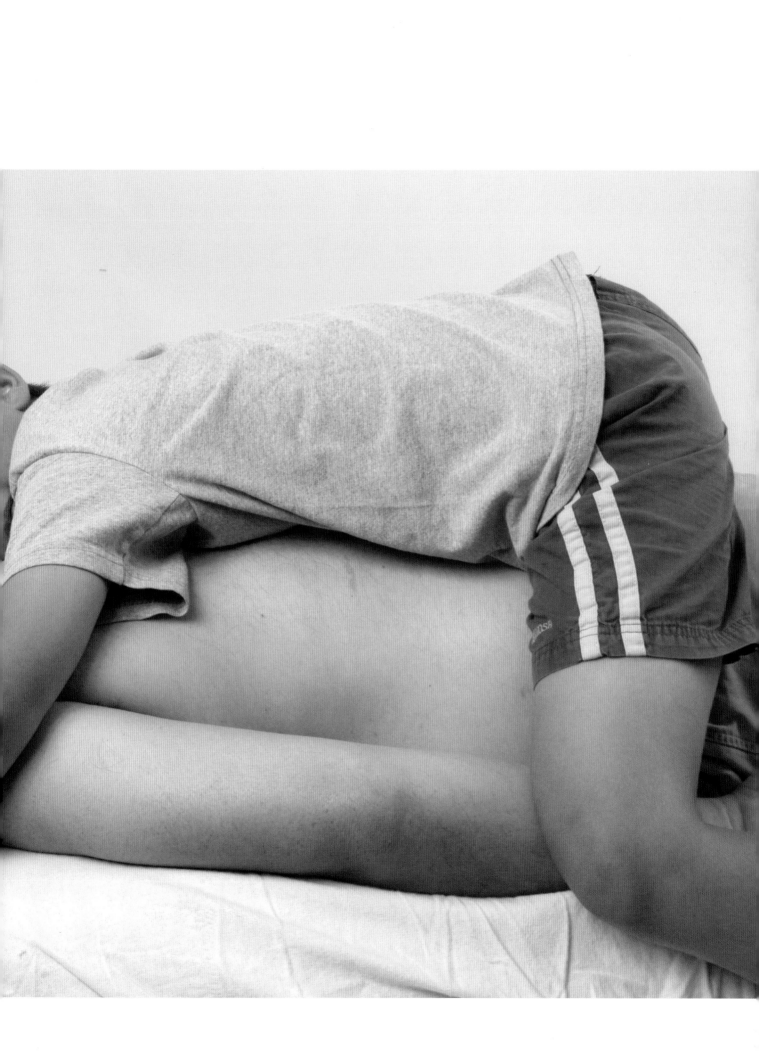

# A HAPPY FAMILY LIFE

A Gallup poll asked Americans what they wanted the most. One answer dominated the list: "A happy family life." But in our high-tech and fast-paced society, we are often disconnected from those we love the most, making the wish for a happy family life more difficult to realize.

Stress is no longer an occasional event but a way of life. Our lives run "pedal to the metal," often stuck in high gear. Husbands and wives have become strangers in their own homes. Divorce is on the rise. Some children turn to drugs. Others, juggling activities and homework, suffer from stress-related disorders. How do we reverse this strong current of tension and disconnect amid our fast and furious lives?

Could it be that the answer to our modern dilemma is as old as time itself? Touch Communications Home Massage says "YES" and is bringing massage—the oldest healing therapy known to man—back into our daily lives.

To achieve a happy family life, experts agree that we need to communicate with each other more, not only via our speech but also with the healing vocabulary of loving touch. Touch is our first language. Whatever our age or stage in life, the gift of touch can make us feel protected, appreciated, and validated, letting us know that we are loved, understood, and forgiven. Home massage brings this healing gift into our homes.

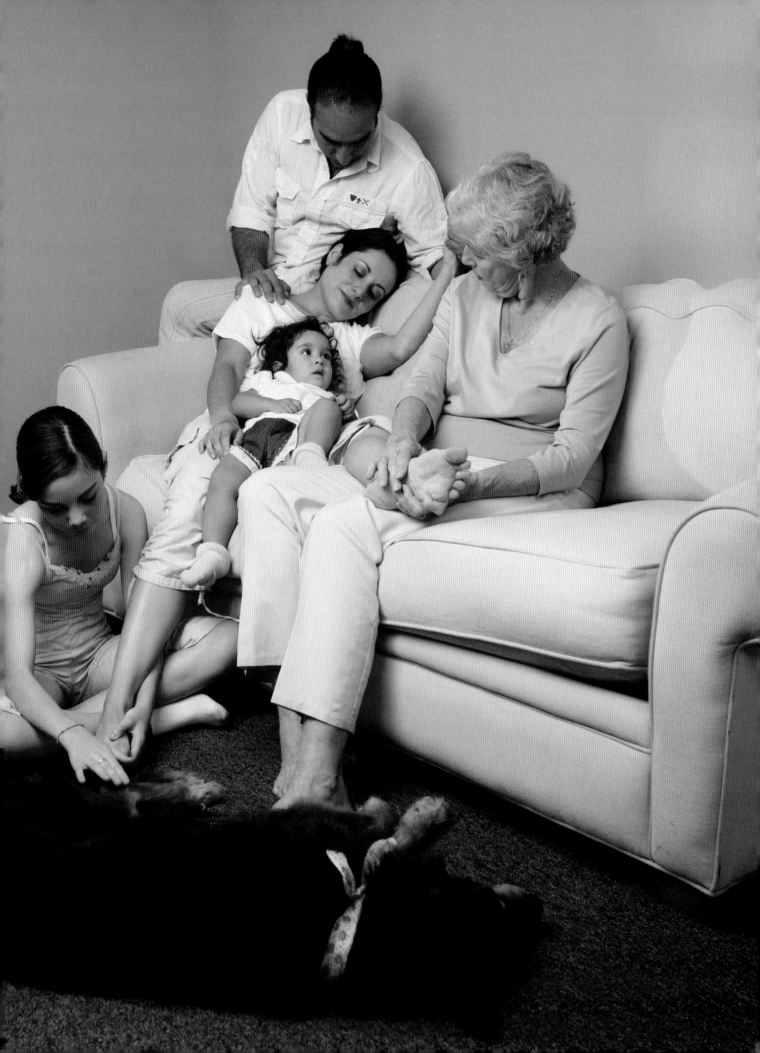

# WHAT BETTER PLACE THAN IN OUR HOME?

There is a resistance in many of us to learning and practicing massage at home. We will nod and agree that it is a great idea. We may even acknowledge the many benefits to both the giver and the receiver. Yet we also feel a certain reluctance to touch.

Maybe in childhood we were never touched, and so massage feels foreign and uncomfortable. What better place than in our own home with the people we love and trust for us to discover and share the healing benefits of touch?

Maybe in childhood we were touched the wrong way, and now we are afraid the same thing will happen again. What better place than a private and safe home environment to heal through the loving, appropriate touch of someone we trust?

Maybe we tell ourselves that we don't have time because of our busy, hectic lives. But home massage is easy and can be done in the convenience of our home. Massage, shared with our loved ones, brings us calm, balance, and an opportunity to rest and recharge from our stressful lives.

Maybe we are uncomfortable with our bodies. We think we are too fat or too thin. We don't want to feel vulnerable. What better place than in our own home to begin to feel at ease with our own unique bodies and so gain a sense of comfort in our own skin?

Maybe we are uncertain how to teach our children about proper and improper touch. What better place than in our home, through shared massage, to open the lines of communication and make touch a household word and natural part of our vocabulary?

Maybe we are too uncomfortable touching another person. With home massage, we can finally give loving touch to our trusted friends and family. Nurturing massage is a gift of healing. What better place than in our own home to share this natural connection with each other?

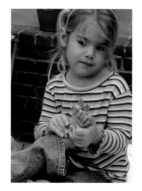

# OUR HOME IS WHERE WE FIRST LEARN TO TOUCH

Massage is now accepted by the general public and the medical community as an valuable adjunct to effective health care. Certified massage therapists with hundreds of hours of training and years of experience are providing relaxation and rehabilitation to everyone from infants to the elderly. But by limiting massage to our infrequent visits to professional massage therapists, the many healing gifts of massage are sadly under-used. Now the healing benefits of massage—stress reduction, pain management, improved immunity, and emotional well-being—are in our hands through home massage.

Home massage, done with the people we already know and trust, is fun, easy to learn, and effective. Home massage is based on three important, tried-and-true principles: creating a safe place of honor and respect, encouraging the art of massage, and taking the mystique out of massage techniques. Following these principles returns us to our natural ability of healing touch. With home massage, the healing benefits of massage are not confined to a massage table. There are a myriad of applications in our daily life for people of all ages and all situations to connect with each other through the art and techniques of home massage.

Massage gives us a way to experience touch for a long enough duration to allow healing of unlimited potential. As insurance and medical costs rise, home massage is an excellent hands-on technique that allows us to take responsibility for our own health and reduce our need for doctors and drugs.

Home is where we first learn to touch, and yet touch is often a neglected means of communication with our family members. When touch through massage becomes a regular and natural part of family life, touch becomes a household word. Parents feel comfortable talking to their children about improper touch and children become receptive and willing to be part of the discussion. Families learn to honor and respect each other through their experience with home massage and report fewer fights, less time watching television, improved health, increased relaxation and renewed emotional connection.

When words fall short, when words can't soothe, and when words are not enough, the power of touch through massage can heal your mind, body, and spirit. We encourage you to learn Touch Communications Home Massage. Experience it. Allow the magic of healing touch to weave into the very fabric of your life. You will be glad you did.

## Authors' note

Although the authors have made every effort to ensure the accuracy and completeness of information contained in this book, we assume no responsibility for errors, inaccuracies, omissions, or any inconsistency herein. Any slights of people, places, or organizations are unintentional.

## Publisher's note

This book is not intended as guidance for the treatment of serious health problems. The information provided is intended to educate and complement, not replace, the advice of your physician or other healthcare professional. Prior to massaging anyone, refer to page 78 for contraindications. Please consult a medical professional if you suffer from any health problems or special conditions.

# UNDERSTANDING HOME MASSAGE

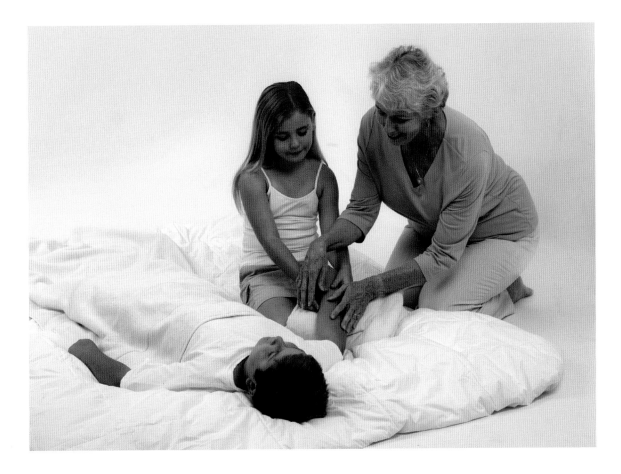

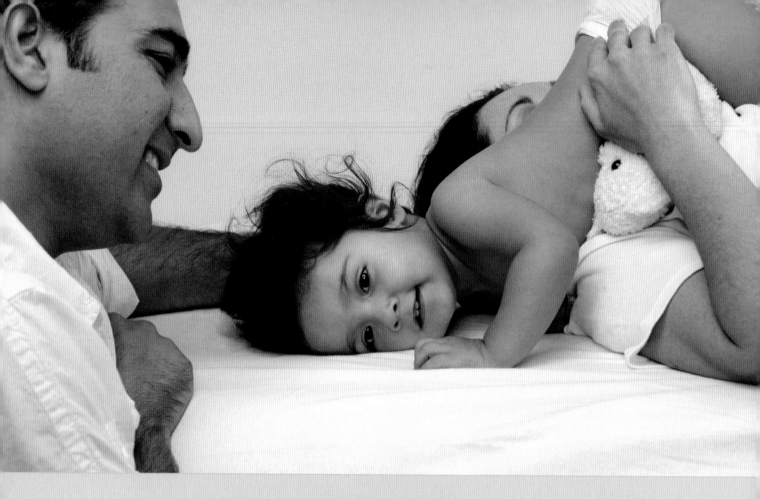

## CHAPTER ONE

# TOUCH HEALS

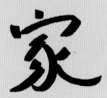

I know that touching was and still is and always will be
the true revolution.

—Nikki Giovanni

Where touching begins, there love and humanity also begin.

—Ashley Montague

# OUR NATURAL INSTINCT

To touch, to hold, and to hug with kindness and compassion are universal and natural instincts. When we gently rub the tired shoulders of a friend, when we embrace, or when we reach out to hold a loved one's hand in kindness and compassion, we are doing something as ancient as time itself.

Touch calms us. It naturally heals us. It makes us feel safe. It makes us feel loved and loving.

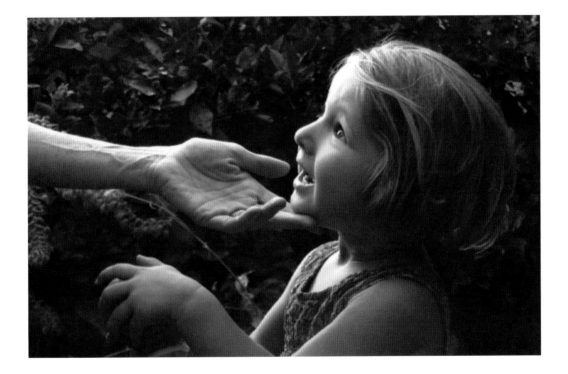

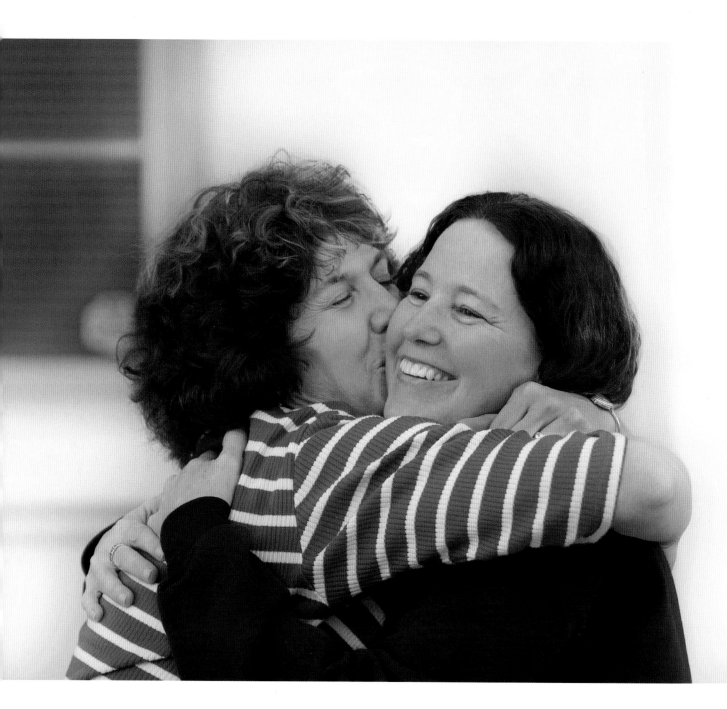

There is nothing that treats our emotional and physical wounds
as much as the bandage of a hug.

# YESTERDAY

Touch is not something we need to learn; it is something we need to remember. The healing power of touch through the art of massage is one of the first healing therapies known to man. Before the advent of drugs, medicine consisted mainly of touch. The earliest tribal cultures throughout the world used touch to cure the sick. To the ancient Greek and Roman physicians, massage was one of the principal means of healing and relieving pain. The "laying on of hands" has been a primary form of healing throughout history. The father of medicine, Hippocrates, wrote, "Physicians must be experienced in many things, but assuredly in rubbing."

# TODAY

Touch is a primal need. It is considered stronger than verbal or emotional contact. Our need and desire for touch is the key to our species, to continuing parenthood, and the survival of the human race. Beyond mere survival, touch improves our physical health, relationships, and emotional well-being.

Today our high-tech and fast-paced lives propel us into an increasingly impersonal world. The detached state of our society is but a reflection of our own individual failure to touch. Virtual reality, chat rooms, and computer games are on the rise and scouting programs, sports leagues, and community groups are on the decline. Sometimes we are more connected to the computer than to our loved ones. The cold metal and hard plastic of our cell phones and iPods has begun to replace the soft, warm touch of those most dear to us.

Living life at high speed also makes it difficult to find the time to connect with those closest to us and maintain our cherished relationships. Gandhi wrote, "There is more to life than increasing its speed." The debris left behind in the whirlwind of our manic desire to get the most done in the least amount of time is ill health and estrangement from family and friends.

Our deep primal need to be touched is even more important today. Our fingertips on a computer may make us feel connected to cyberspace, but the same hands placed upon a loved one can give the gift of healing, connection, and relaxation. The power of touch through home massage can return balance, health, and calm to our often hectic and impersonal lives.

# RESEARCH STUDIES ON TOUCH

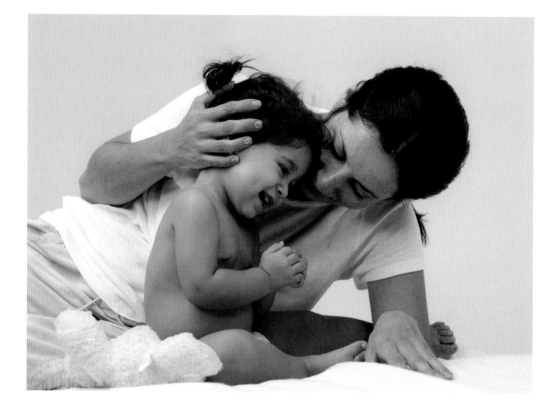

Landmark research on touch with rhesus monkeys shows they prefer surrogate mother objects providing contact comfort (frames covered with terry cloth) to those consisting of frames with bare wires that provide a steady milk supply. This reveals that it is touch, not food, that promotes the greater attachment.[1]

Longitudinal studies of rhesus monkeys also indicate that touch deprivation has an impact on physiological functions, such as stress hormone response and immunological strength.[2]

Recent research in humans shows that aberrant behavior stemming from early touch deprivation is sustained, repeated, and reinforced from generation to generation.[3,4]

A research study of 49 cultures revealed that those exhibiting minimal physical affection towards their children had significantly higher rates of violence. Those that showed the most amounts of physical affection had the least occurrence of adult violence.[5]

A study examining the effects of massage on women receiving massage (30-minute massage three times weekly for five weeks) showed reduced anxiety, depressed mood and anger. The longer-term massage effects included reduced depression and hostility, increased urinary dopamine, serotonin values, natural killer cell number and lymphocytes.[6]

In a study on HIV-positive adults, natural killer cells increased after 20 days of massage.[7]

After five weeks of twice-weekly massages, adults with spinal cord injuries saw their functional activity improve and experienced increased range of motion in their wrists and elbows.[8]

Short sessions of soft-tissue massage provided a sense of meaning and inner respite among cancer patients in palliative care, according to recent research.[9]

Research studies concluded that therapeutic massage was an effective treatment providing long-lasting benefits for patients suffering from chronic low back pain. Researchers hypothesize that massage might be an effective alternative to conventional medical care for persistent low back pain.[10]

A pilot study revealed that massage reduces pain and muscle spasms in patients who have undergone heart bypass surgery when patients are treated with massage at the hospital after their surgery. Because of its effectiveness, 60 percent of the massage group expressed a willingness to pay for massage therapy out-of-pocket.[11]

Furthermore, research studies have found that massage is helpful in decreasing blood pressure in people with hypertension, alleviating pain in migraine sufferers, and improving alertness and performance in office workers.[12]

# TOUCHY ABOUT TOUCH

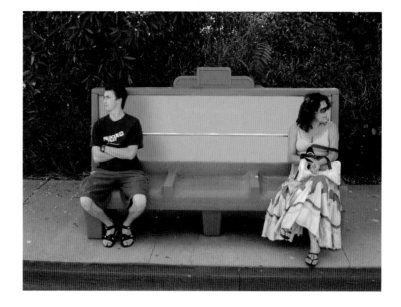

Research has now proven what the ancients always knew—touch heals. Ironically, the high-tech world that created the equipment to scientifically reveal the healing power of touch is "out of touch" with touch.

In the United States, we are usually at the forefront of new ideas. But, unfortunately, our society has become touch-phobic. America is what anthropologists call a "non-tactile society." Compared with most societies around the world, we are "touchy about touch." Sadly, our attitudes about touch are influenced by our culture and not our need for touch. Our culture has now convinced us that touch is dangerous. Fears of sexual abuse and improper touch haunt innocent adults. No-touch laws in schools restrict teachers from hugging their students or even picking up preschoolers who fall on the playground. Many parents are confused about how and where to touch their children. Others wonder, "How old is too old to touch?"

The truth is that we have become a "touch-starved" nation. We hunger for touch and connection with the people in our lives. Many people are unaware of the emotional and physical effects of their touch deprivation. Some adults unconsciously develop psychosomatic illnesses in hopes of receiving the gentle, nurturing touch they remember from childhood. The elderly often ask others to take their hand, not for stability, but because they crave touch. Children pretend to be sick, not necessarily to stay home from school as parents suspect, but to receive their healing touch and attention.

Sometimes we go to great lengths to show friends and family we care about them through giving or doing, but we are reluctant to embrace them.

Secretly a mother would like to express affection to her teenage son. Secretly he would enjoy it—just as he did in childhood—but instead he snarls, "Leave me alone!"

A father, leaving on a trip, starts to kiss his daughter goodbye but is hurt when she turns and gives him an uncomfortable shrug instead.

A small child deliberately disobeys his parent for the payoff of being spanked. To some children, negative touch is better than no touch at all.

We visit a relative in the hospital, bringing flowers and candy, but we may be reluctant to give them a healing hug or to hold their hand.

A grieving friend needs a compassionate hug, but we are uncomfortable and so offer only awkward words of condolence.

We intuitively know that touch is healing, but sometimes we fear the honesty of touch. The truth is that often touch is more than appropriate—it may be the very best way to communicate and connect with those we love.

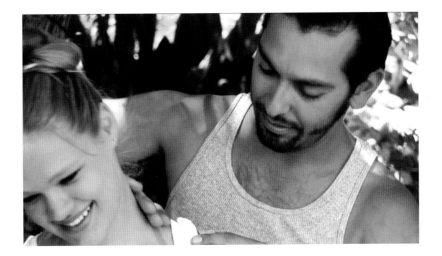

# PROPER TOUCH

Touch, like fire, can hurt or heal you.

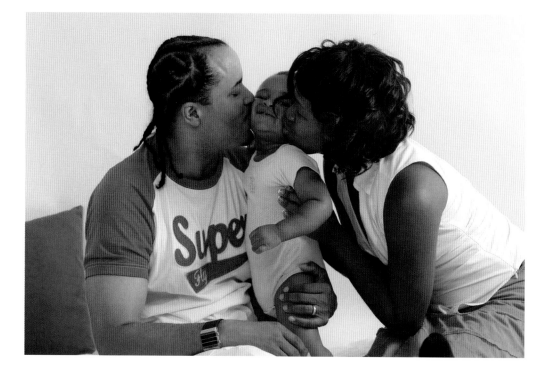

Touch can be a healing gift or a damaging poison. Children have been wounded with life-long scars from the devastating effects of abusive touch. Bad touch makes us feel uncomfortable, scared, nervous, and threatened. Healing touch makes us feel comfortable, calm, peaceful, and safe.

We face the dilemma of knowing that touch is critical for our health and well-being, but that improper touch can scar our very soul. And so a great schism divides our culture: to touch or not to touch?

If we choose not to touch, we are robbing ourselves and future generations of one of our most precious birthrights—the innate healing power of touch. The art of massage, shared between family and friends whom we love and trust, can help us reclaim that deep heritage of healing touch for ourselves and our children.

# TO TOUCH OR NOT TO TOUCH

There is nothing more hideous,
More damaging,
More disappointing,
Than the touch that shatters our trust.
It can break our heart;
It can reach our core;
It can scar our soul.


There is nothing more accessible,
More under-used,
More needed,
More healing,
Than sacred touch.
It can mend a broken heart;
It can make us feel more alive;
It can refresh our mind;
It can soothe our soul.

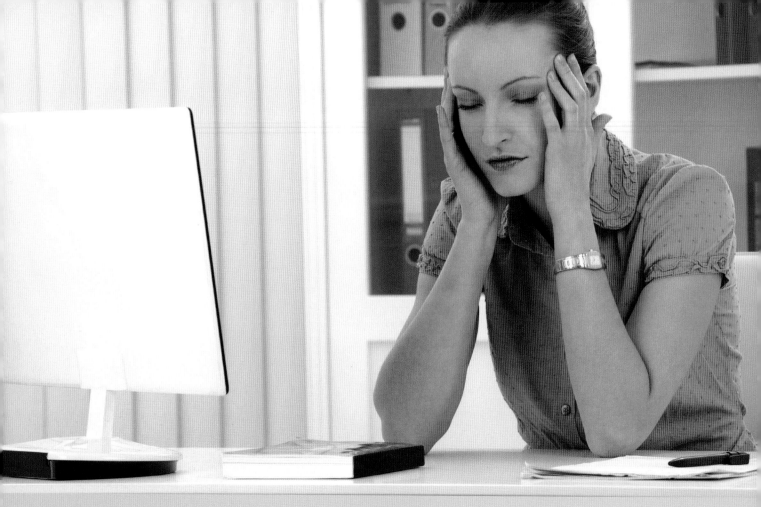

CHAPTER TWO

# S T R E S S

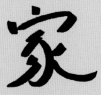

The time to relax is when you don't have time to relax.

All this talk and turmoil and noise and movement is outside
the veil. Inside the veil is silence and calm and peace
~Bayazid Bistami

# STRESS KILLS

Our bodies have forgotten how relaxation feels. We have come to accept our fast-paced, over-loaded, and increasingly impersonal lives as normal. As self-help author and motivational speaker Richard Carlson states, "Stress is nothing more than a socially acceptable form of mental illness."

Stress can be seductive and strong, dominating our lives and luring us in with the adrenaline rush of life on full throttle. Too much to do with too little time is our national anthem. Some label it the American Way or modern living. But perhaps it is our collective insanity that has us all convinced that our exhaustion from competing demands, overabundant choices, and over-extended schedules is either natural or impossible to avoid.

Stress is the gradual and insidious running down of our general health. Outside pressures such as work, family tensions, and bad nutrition take their toll on our mind, body and spirit. Stress can also emanate from inside us through negative thoughts, constant worrying and low self-esteem. No matter what the gender, economic status, or position, no one is immune from the damaging effects of stress. Chronic stress undermines the body's ability to fix itself and causes psychological and physical disease. We can hardly pick up a newspaper or watch television without seeing and hearing about a new study relating stress to a variety of illnesses. A public health survey estimated that 70 to 80 percent of Americans who visit conventional physicians suffer from stress-related or "lifestyle" diseases. Perhaps the most damaging effect of stress is that we have lost touch with just how much this chronic tension is controlling our relationships, our physical health, and our emotional well-being.

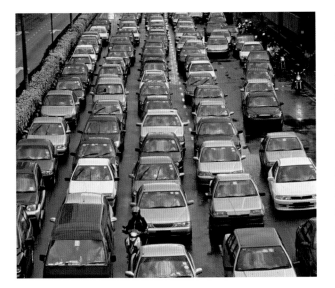

Consider stress on the freeway. If you want to break it down to what the cell understands, it is chemical stress because of the smog. Being on the freeway is emotional stress because you are not happy to be there. Being on the freeway is structural stress because your heart and lungs and kidneys don't function as well when you are cramped up in your tight little car seat.

—Dr. Vincent Medici

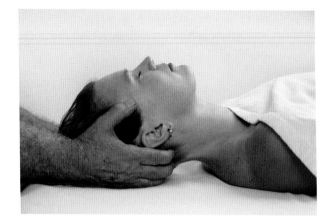

*Stress is an ignorant state.*
*It believes that everything is an emergency.*

—Natalie Goldberg

## SYMPTOMS OF STRESS

Heart Disease

Infections

Poor Immunity

Eating Disorders

High Blood Pressure

Migraines

Gastrointestinal Distress

Muscular Pain

Loneliness

Depression

Tight Muscles

Memory Loss

Sleep Disturbances

Racing Heart

Sexual Dysfunction

Fatigue

Mental Illness

Ulcers

Diabetes

Low Back Pain

Substance Abuse

Shortness of Breath

# THE STRESS RESPONSE
## FIGHT OR FLIGHT
### The Sympathetic Nervous System

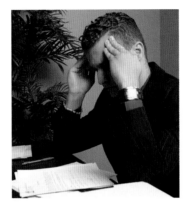

The stress response is our body's rapid and automatic switch into high gear. During the stress response our body is like a plane readying itself for take-off. Our heart, blood, lungs, digestion, and brain are all activated and set to go. This reaction helps us deal with physical threats by giving us more energy, speed, concentration, and agility to protect ourselves or to run as fast as possible. But physical threats aren't the only events that trigger this stress response. Psychological threats—pressures at work, interpersonal issues, money worries, illness, or the death of a loved one—can also set off the same alarm system. Even the typical day-to-day demands of living can contribute to our body's stress response.

Any situation that we perceive as dangerous, even subconsciously or falsely, is experienced as a threat to our sympathetic nervous system. Our bodies react by prompting our adrenal glands to release a series of stress hormones, adrenaline and cortisol, increasing our heart rate, elevating our blood pressure, and boosting our energy.

Under most circumstances, once the acute threat has passed our relaxation response returns all systems to neutral. But modern life poses ongoing stressful situations that are not short-lived, creating chronic stress. Thus we run on a fight-or-flight reaction longer than is necessary or healthy.

What is good for the body on a short-term basis can be very harmful over long periods of time. A nervous system under chronic stress can, as a result, either become hyperactive (frenetic) or hypoactive (underactive). The disharmony of these two natural and essential forces can then imbalance many of our physiological activities and contribute to, or create, various physical and psychological conditions.

Our bodies have forgotten
how relaxation feels.

Massage returns us to our
natural, calm state of being.

# THE STRESS RESPONSE
## REST AND DIGEST
### The Parasympathetic Nervous System

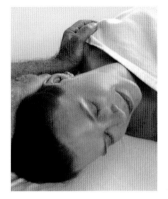

How we perceive a stress-provoking event will determine its impact on our health. Not all stressful situations are negative. The birth of a child, a job promotion, or a new relationship may not be perceived as dangerous to our body. However, we may feel that these situations are stressful because they are new or we are not fully prepared to deal with them.

Perhaps nothing can age us more rapidly—internally and externally—than high stress. Unfortunately, when we are under stress it is difficult for us to maintain the habits that lead to a healthy life. Instead of exercising, some people respond by inactivity and overeating. Instead of eating healthy, we succumb to increasingly poor nutritional choices. Instead of practicing moderation, we abuse alcohol, smoke, and self-medicate.

Although stress is a fact of life, steps can be taken to manage the impact that life events have on you. First, learn to identify stressful events and develop healthy ways of dissipating this daily strain, such as exercise, healthy eating, social support, and psychotherapy. Add to that regular massage, which can be very effective in balancing the nervous system and restoring homeostasis (physical balance and equilibrium). The skin and muscles contain many nerve endings and connections. The soothing, balancing, healing touch of massage is relayed by them to every part of the body to bring relief and promote well-being.

Touch Communications Home Massage is an excellent method you can bring into your daily life to alleviate tension and remind the body how relaxation feels. There is no single cure-all, but integrating home massage into your life can help you manage stress, connect with the people you love, create a peaceful home environment, and help you enjoy a longer, healthier life.

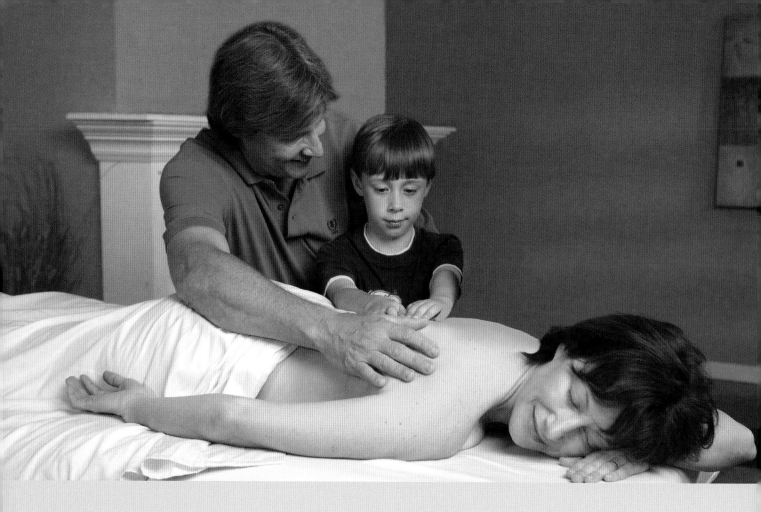

## CHAPTER THREE

# HOME MASSAGE

Touch is a path to peace in our world.
It is the realization of the
oneness of humanity.

What better place
than in our home,
through the universal language of touch,
to plant the seeds of peace?

— *Jackie Sloan*

# MASSAGE HEALS

Massage is good medicine. Americans make 60 million visits to massage practitioners every year. Massage is now recognized by both the medical community and the public as an integral part of health care. Some insurance companies offer reimbursement for massage to treat various ailments. Infant massage is on the rise and is being taught to parents around the country. Instead of coffee breaks or two-martini lunches, many companies offer chair massages during the lunch hour as part of their wellness program. Hospitals are introducing massage for their patients to reduce pain, alleviate anxiety, and boost their immune systems. Recognizing that healing, caring touch is good for everyone, community centers and colleges around the nation are offering massage classes to teach the general public how to give an effective massage.

Professional massage therapists are well educated with hundreds of hours of classes and years of training in a variety of modalities such as Trager, Rolfing, cranial sacral, and polarity bodywork. Their sincere desire to help others, combined with their specialized expertise, allows them to effectively treat a variety of physical and emotional ailments, offering an invaluable contribution to our health care system. Trained massage therapists now work in hospitals, psychiatric units, rehabilitation centers, special-care baby units, nursing homes, and medical centers. Anyone who has ever gone to a certified massage therapist for assistance with anything from stress reduction to specific injuries knows the value of a professional massage.

Factors of cost and convenience can limit visits to certified massage therapists, and thus we are vastly underutilizing the many healing benefits of massage. The truth is that you don't have to be a massage therapist to give a soothing, healing massage. Anyone can do it. The benefits of massage—reducing stress, soothing overworked muscles, boosting our immune system, and meeting our emotional needs for touch— are in our own hands. When massage is done in the comfort and familiarity of our homes with the people we already trust and respect, we feel safe, allowing the magic of massage to happen with very little effort.

With home massage, we find relief from a variety of ailments without the financial burden of medical bills. As health insurance costs soar, our need for self-responsibility and prevention becomes even more important. The health care of the future will include effective, low-cost interventions like home massage used side by side with sophisticated new techniques. Hands-on healing will help lessen our need for doctor visits, drugs and hospital care. The convenience of home massage makes it a valuable tool that can be used with almost limitless frequency. It can aid in not only the treatment but in the prevention of so many ailments of daily life—everything from sports injuries to pain management to stress reduction. It can promote relaxation and, ultimately, our emotional well-being.

# HEALING BENEFITS
# OF HOME MASSAGE

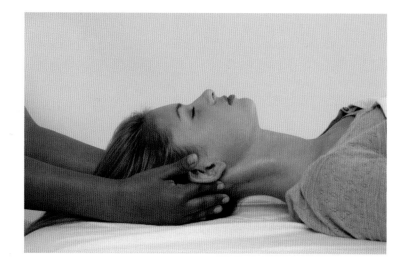

Relaxes the nervous system, relieving anxiety, lifting depression, and boosting energy.

Increases joint flexibility and relaxes and softens injured and overused muscles.

Creates a relaxed state of being. Regular sessions significantly reduce stress.

Brings awareness of our mind-body connection.

Assists the blood flow, encourages the lymphatic drainage, and stretches the connective tissue of our joints.

Boosts our immune system.

Improves circulation, bringing much needed oxygen and other nutrients to our tissue.

Fulfills our emotional need for caring, nurturing touch.

Releases endorphins, the body's natural painkiller.

# THE MAGIC
# OF HOME MASSAGE

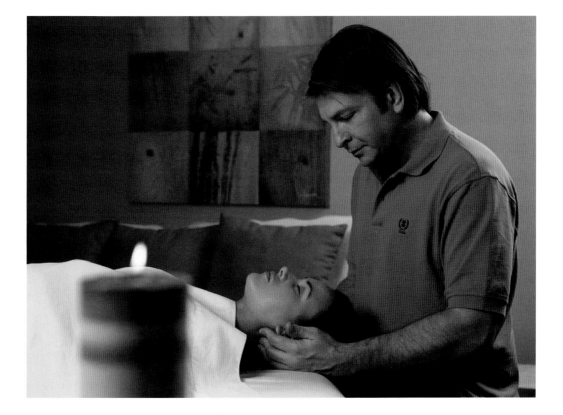

The magic of home massage comes from not only the quality of touch but also the duration. Where else but through massage can we touch each other in a healing, comfortable, and nonsexual way for one minute, five minutes, 30 minutes, or an hour? The real benefits of massage for both the giver and receiver are realized with the duration of touch. This is where the magic happens. Massage opens the door and gives us a safe and concrete way to touch our partners in a loving, nurturing way for a sufficient amount of time to make the cells in our body happy, excited, fulfilled and healthy.

When we become comfortable massaging someone—when we can give and receive non-sexual touch for 10 to 50 minutes—we are transformed. Translated to our everyday lives, we are able to keep that 20-second hug going for 35 seconds, hold the hand of a sick relative for two full minutes and hug our son or daughter when it previously felt uncomfortable. Through home massage, we return to our innate ability for and comfort with healing touch.

# FAMILY CONNECTION

*A family in harmony will prosper in everything.*
—Chinese proverb

*Home is where one starts from.*
—T. S. Eliot

No other institution in our society does more than a loving family to shape our values, support our needs, and nurture our mind, body, and spirit. The family provides not only food and shelter, but also love, security, and a sense of belonging. What we learn or don't learn from our family can affect us for a lifetime, shaping who we are, how we live, and how we interact with the world. A strong family is our anchor in a world that is inherently unpredictable and constantly changing.

Our first experience with touch is our mother's loving caress in our home. Within our family we learn how, when and where to touch. Yet natural touch among family members is an often neglected means of communication. Touch is vital to our relationships. It is critical for our growth and development. It is essential to our emotional well-being. What better place than within our family to rediscover the healing benefits of touch? And what better way than through the medium of massage to express loving touch to those closest to us?

When the massage table becomes as natural a piece of furniture as the living room sofa, families achieve better health, increased relaxation, and a deeper connection with each other. Parents have a way to relieve stress and enjoy renewed intimacy. Children fight less as they learn to nurture each other. When massage is a natural routine, families learn to express themselves easily through the language of touch, creating harmony, mutual respect, and stability in our homes.

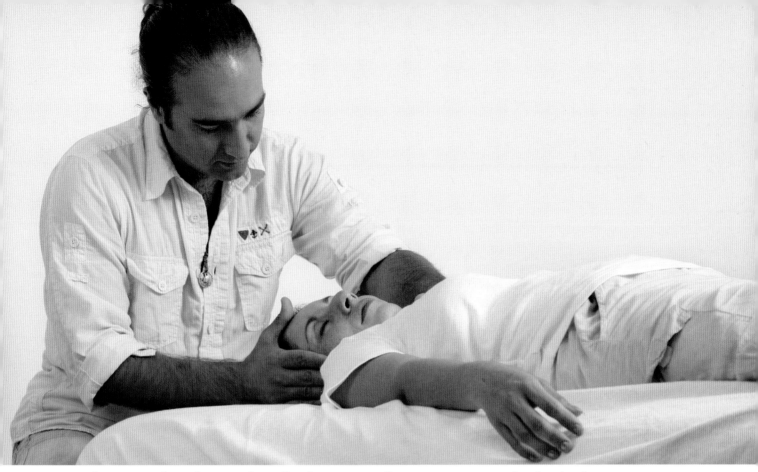

Time alone together sharing the gift of massage allows every pair in the family the opportunity
to connect with the opening of the heart and the relaxing of the ego.
The giver becomes the receiver and the receiver becomes the giver.
And, in that special moment, they become one.

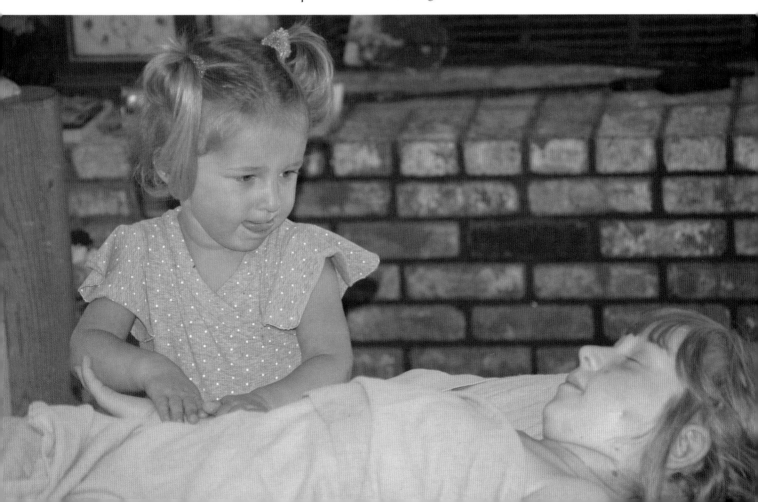

# HOME MASSAGE MAKES TOUCH A HOUSEHOLD WORD

There is no place like home.

—Dorothy, *The Wizard of Oz*

What better place than in our own homes to regain our comfort with touch? Fears and inhibitions about touch begin in our home, but they can also end there. Home massage makes touch a household word instead of allowing it to become a taboo subject. Too often parents, in an attempt to protect their children from the dangers of improper touch, are reluctant to discuss issues surrounding touch or, even worse, they discourage any kind of touch. Often they wait until their children are teenagers, unwilling to listen and thus more influenced by their peers. Adults who are raised in families where touch was awkward or discouraged often suffer from a discomfort with touch that can affect their relationships in ways both disguised and apparent.

When massage is part of our daily lives, it becomes a natural bridge for both adults and children to talk easily about issues relating to touch. Home massage reminds us that our bodies belong to us. Through exchanging massage with our loved ones, we learn to communicate what kind of pressure we want, where we want to be massaged, and when something doesn't feel good. The trust and comfort that grows on the massage table can easily be transferred to more delicate and personal matters. By experiencing loving, safe, and appropriate touch, we also learn to understand the many signs our bodies offer us when touched appropriately. Furthermore, the confidence gained on the massage table will help us recognize the signs and communicate our concerns when touch is not appropriate.

Once we become comfortable with touch on the massage table, we don't need to be told how to touch, where to touch, what is bad touch, or be convinced of our need to be touched. We experience a return to our natural expression of touch. As touch becomes a household word through massage, everyone learns to honor and respect themselves and each other in all matters of touch.

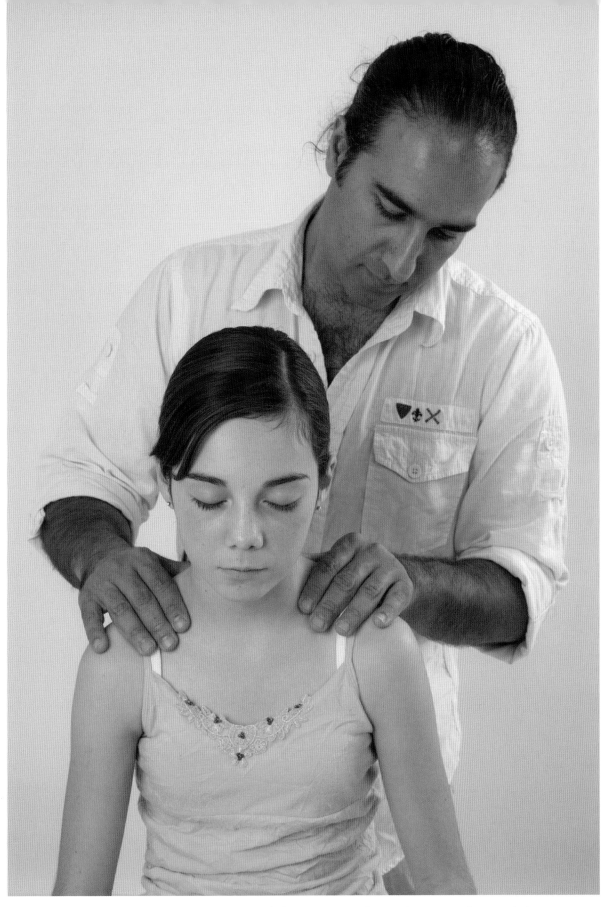

Fears and inhibitions about touch begin in our home but can also end there.

# LEARNING
# HOME MASSAGE

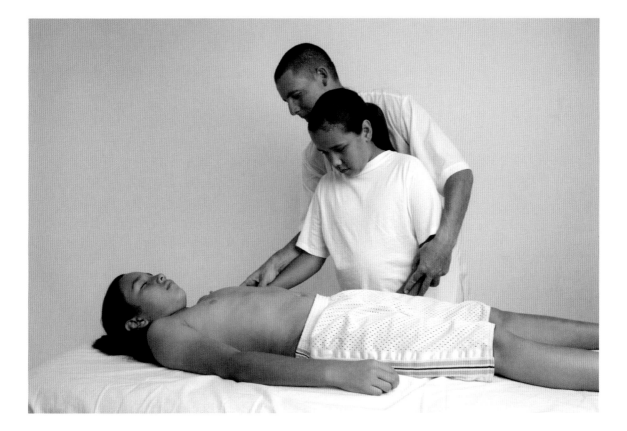

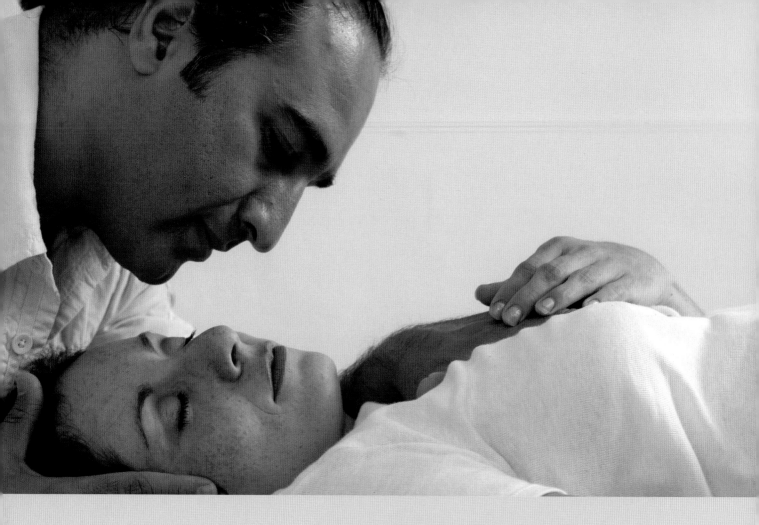

CHAPTER FOUR

# THE
# THREE PRINCIPLES
## OF TOUCH COMMUNICATIONS HOME MASSAGE

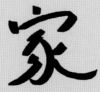

In the beginner's mind there are many possibilities,
but in the expert's there are few.

—Shunryu Suzuki

You don't have to be a massage therapist to give a good massage. Anyone can do it. The tried and true principles of TCHM are a winning formula that makes massage easy and fun to learn. Use these three simple but powerful principles and you will naturally return to your innate ability for healing touch.

# PRINCIPLE ONE

## CREATE A SAFE PLACE
## OF HONOR AND RESPECT

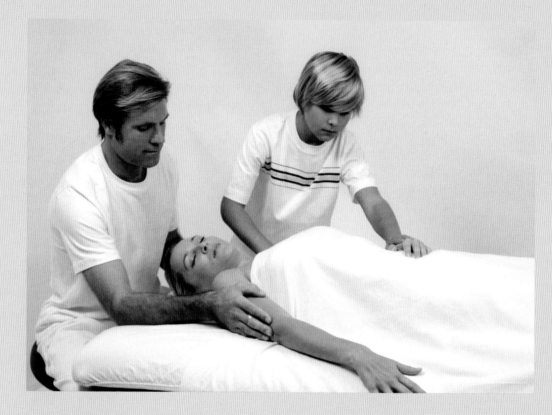

When the recipient of massage feels safe, that person is able to relax and the magic of massage happens with very little effort. This applies to anyone we are massaging—young or old, family member or trusted friend. The beauty of home massage is that by working on family and friends, a certain level of trust already exists, allowing relaxation to occur at a deeper level. Understanding that we are creating a sacred, safe place of honor and respect builds upon that trust and allows for deep healing.

# LEARN TO LISTEN

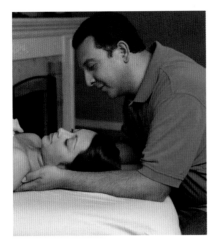

Massage is a conversation without words. Listening to the person on the table with your whole mind, body, and spirit takes energy and the best of intentions. Just as we practice our massage techniques, we should also continually practice listening. How well we listen to what is happening beneath our hands resonates with the receiver and either takes them deeper into, or further away from, a state of relaxation and peace.

If the receiver asks you to turn the music down and you don't oblige, he or she will feel slighted. If the receiver asks you not to massage a certain part of their body and you do anyway, they will not feel safe. If a spouse even jokingly makes an unkind remark towards their mate, their body will become tense.

Occasionally, during or after a massage, the receiver may verbally share something personal with the giver. It is natural, especially between family and friends, to want to help and so the temptation might be to lecture or give advice. Good listening, without offering advice, makes the receiver feel safe and accepted versus judged and analyzed. Always remember the tremendous healing power of simply listening.

## AN UNWRITTEN CONTRACT

The giver creates an unwritten contract with the receiver that the massage will be done with a great sense of honor and respect. There is an agreement that the massage is a "time out" from our daily responsibilities and there will be no talk about such things as money, school or work.

There is an agreement that the massage will be nonsexual in conversation, insinuation, and behavior.

Both the giver and receiver will enter the massage with a kind, patient, and nonjudgmental spirit.

When the unwritten contract is understood and consistently experienced, trust grows and the receiver will let go and a healing, relaxing massage will naturally occur.

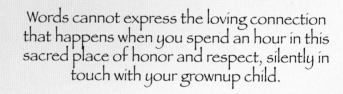

Words cannot express the loving connection
that happens when you spend an hour in this
sacred place of honor and respect, silently in
touch with your grownup child.

# HONOR YOURSELF

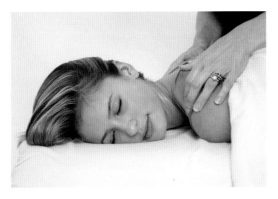

The benefits of home massage go far beyond the massage session. The lessons learned from the first principle can also improve our daily lives.

It is just as important for the receiver to communicate when they don't like the way they are being touched as when they are enjoying a certain technique. When receiving a massage, clearly communicate to the giver when something feels uncomfortable or inappropriate. We've all had experiences when someone has violated our boundaries, whether by a family member, friend, relative, or co-worker. What do we do? Do we let it pass? Do we confront the person? Do we allow it to continue? It is critical for children and adults to be aware of their physical and emotional boundaries. For example, "I don't want my feet massaged," or "Please use a softer touch," or "I want to be fully clothed during the massage."

Creating a safe place of honor and respect means that both the giver and the receiver honor themselves as well as each other. As the giver, never agree to massage someone you are not comfortable touching.

It takes effort and practice to learn to assert ourselves, but it is worth the rewards. Expressing our boundaries during home massage will transfer to other areas of our lives. Real boundaries come from inside as we learn what we want, what is crossing a line, and what signals our bodies offer when touched appropriately and inappropriately. Adopting a healthy attitude about touch teaches our children to honor their bodies. This will do more to prevent improper touch than instilling fear and avoidance.

## COMPASSIONATE TOUCH

Creating a safe place of honor and respect through compassionate, non-judgmental touch allows the receiver to relax, let go, and heal emotionally and physically. The receiver should always feel a deep sense of safety and inner calmness when he or she is on the table. Let your hands be the healing instruments that convey kindness, compassion, and respect .

Everything we do during a massage—putting a bolster under a leg, lifting hair off the face, folding a blanket back, or applying oil—should be done with great care, deliberation and honor.

This principle applies to anyone we are massaging—child, spouse, friend, elderly person, or sibling. Don't assume that because you are familiar with, older than, or a parent of the person on the table that you should relax this principle. The magic of massage happens when you completely honor and respect whomever is on the table.

# PRINCIPLE TWO

## ENCOURAGE THE ART OF MASSAGE

If you want to know what true art is: Go outside on a
clear night, wait until it gets very, very dark, and look
up. You will see no rules of composition, no evidence of
superior technique. Yet you will be staring into the face
of pure, unadulterated beauty and wonder.
—Derek R. Audette

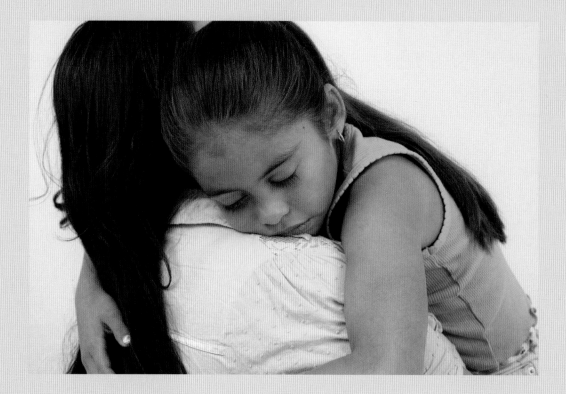

Have you ever been massaged by an electronic massager? Many variations exist in the
marketplace. The mechanics are there but the human touch is absent. Have you ever
been hugged by someone and it somehow felt awkward, preoccupied and without
emotion? Compare that with a hug from a child who is comfortable with touch, gives
you his or her whole attention and whose emotions are pure and spontaneous.

# INTENTIONS

The "art of massage" focuses on being present and being comfortable in mind, body and spirit. The techniques of massage comprise our brush and paints. Our canvas is the receiver of the massage. The art of massage comes from what is within us. It is the way we hold the "brush"—our intentions, our heartfelt presence, and our comfort level—that separates an ordinary massage from a great, healing massage.

# BEING PRESENT

Massage is a meditation shared by two people—a quiet conversation through the medium of touch. Moment to moment, all that should exist for the giver is the comfort, safety, and relaxation of the person on the table. If outside thoughts come, allow them to pass by and then return to your breath and the sensation of the receiver's skin against your hands. Being present in mind, body, and spirit allows you to focus all your energy on the massage.

The dynamics of the giver and receiver relationship should never become a power imbalance that makes the person on the table feel vulnerable. It is critical that the giver of the massage is always present with "good intentions." The vulnerability of the receiver should be met with kindness and compassion. Rather than feeling powerful, he or she should be thankful for the privilege of massaging his or her partner.

# BEING COMFORTABLE

Your comfort as the giver is as important as the comfort of the receiver. A great massage should be as relaxing for the giver as for the person on the table. This is why it is important to find a comfortable place to work. As the giver, keep your body as free from tension as possible. Remember to occasionally bring your attention back to your own level of relaxation to make sure you are not stiffening your body and passing that tension on to the receiver. The more relaxed you are touching your partner, the more comfortable she will be accepting your touch.

Being comfortable will allow the massage to reach another level. If we can be physically and emotionally relaxed when we touch the receiver, she will be able to let go and release tension that resides deep within the body.

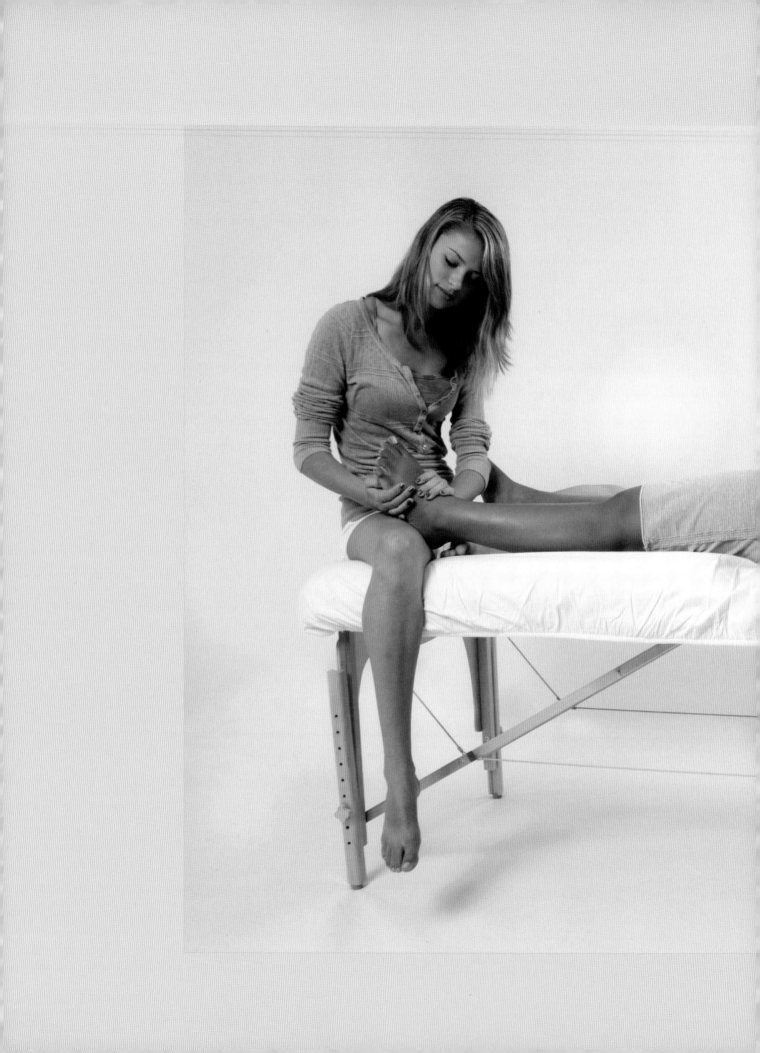

The art of massage is about being comfortable in mind, body and spirit.
When the giver is comfortable it resonates with the receiver
and they naturally relax and heal.

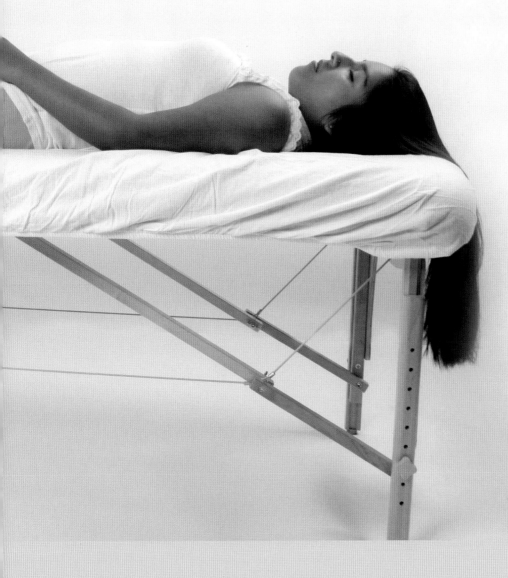

# PRINCIPLE THREE
## TAKE THE MYSTIQUE
## OUT OF MASSAGE TECHNIQUES

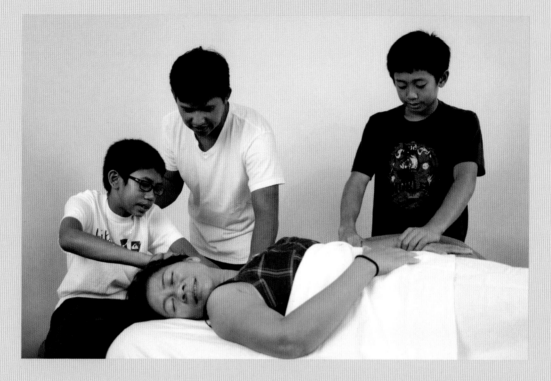

We work with being, but non-being is what we are.
—Lao-Tzu

What is the mystique of massage? It is normal for beginning students to think that massage is about learning a precise way of doing techniques. The misconception is that the larger the arsenal of techniques we have, the better the massage. This is not so.

Massage techniques are important in giving a healing massage. But massage techniques by themselves don't heal. It is the connection between the giver and the receiver during the massage that is the catalyst for healing. Blending techniques with a safe environment and the art of massage creates a healing experience.

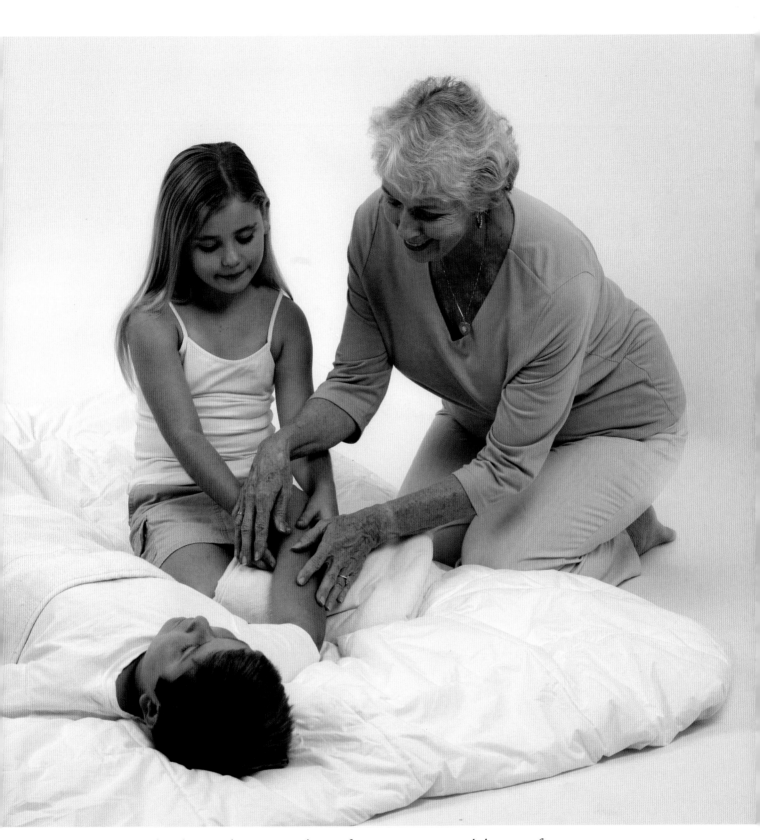

Blending techniques with a safe environment and the art of massage
creates a healing experience.

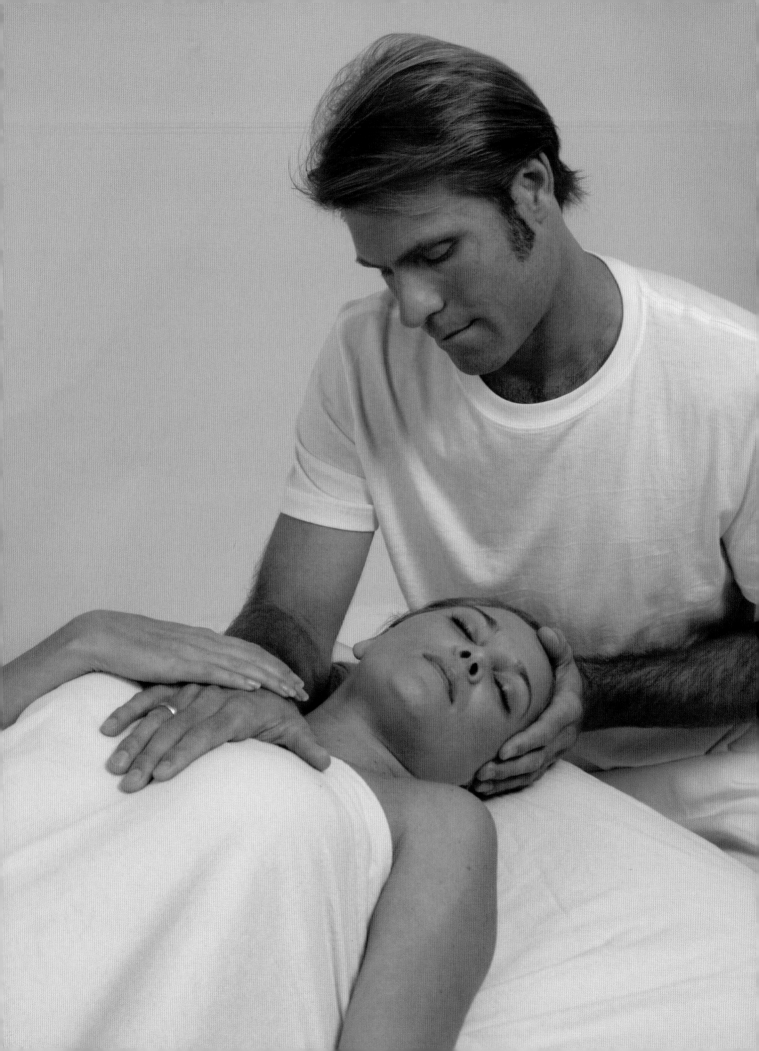

It is the connection between the giver and receiver,
not complicated massage moves, that heals.

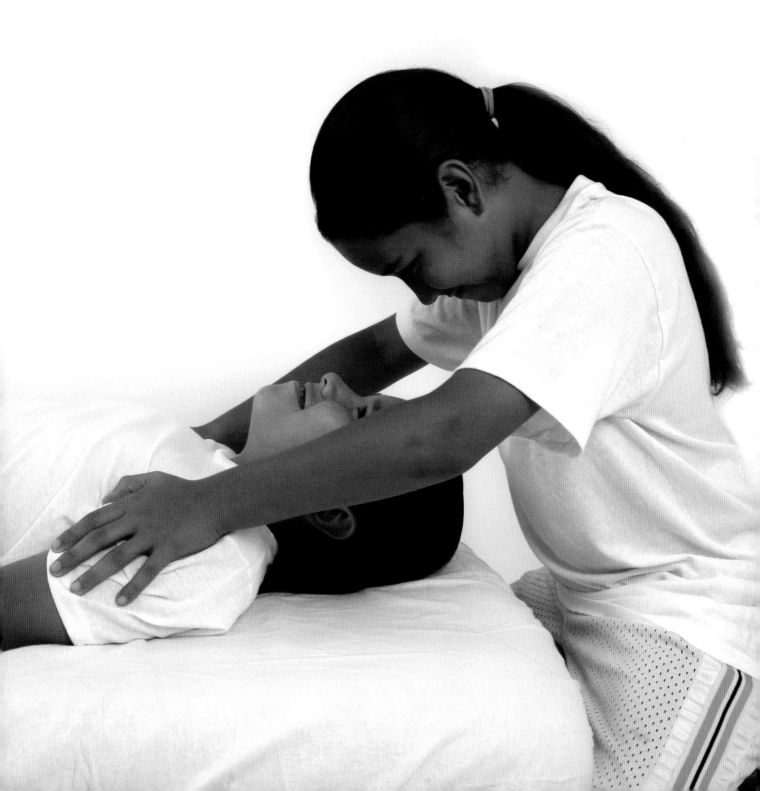

CHAPTER FIVE

# PREPARATION

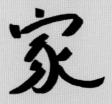

The beauty of Touch Communications Home Massage is that it can be done anywhere and anytime. No specialized equipment is needed—only your healing hands,
your good intentions, and a willing and trusting partner. Our sense of calm and relaxation is affected by the environment that surrounds us. Thus, some forethought in
creating the most comfortable environment for both the giver and the receiver will
greatly enhance a feeling of deep relaxation. Healing takes place when the massage
flows without interruption and distractions.

# THE ROOM

Relaxation is paramount to giving a good massage. Take the time to create a calm and secure space that makes the receiver feel relaxed and comfortable. Provide a quiet, private, uncluttered space away from household distractions. Turn off or disconnect all phones. Make sure that you have enough room to easily move around the table. Keep a good supply of massage oil or lotion close by. It is a good idea to provide a supply of cotton sheets that you use only for massage. Twin size sheets work the best. Flannel sheets provide extra warmth. Have a pillow or bolster for the legs.

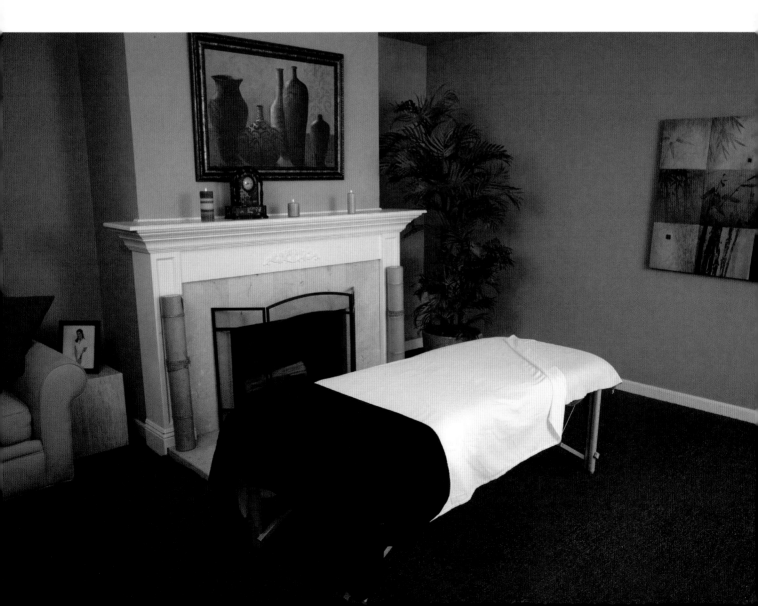

# LIGHTING

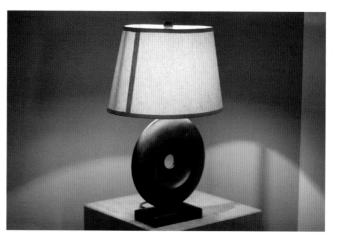

Make sure the lighting is soft and subdued to allow the eyes of the receiver to relax completely. Natural light provides the best atmosphere. Soft lights work when there is no natural light available. Provide a small table lamp or floor lamp away from the massage table. Candles are a nice mood enhancer. Make sure, however, they don't create a fire hazard.

# TEMPERATURE

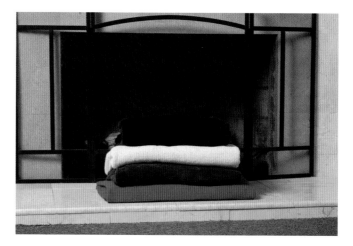

Many people cool down during a massage and get chilled. Provide a room that is warm and draft free. A space heater works well to warm the area around the massage table. Have a blanket nearby to cover your partner.

# TIME

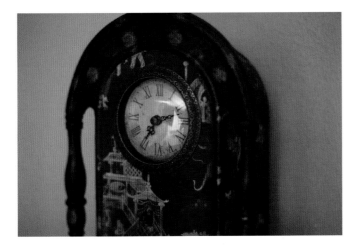

Choose a time when you and your partner will be undisturbed. Relaxation can go deeper and deeper when there are no interruptions. Decide beforehand how long the massage will last. Let others in your household know that this is your time and ask them to honor your space without interruptions.

# MUSIC

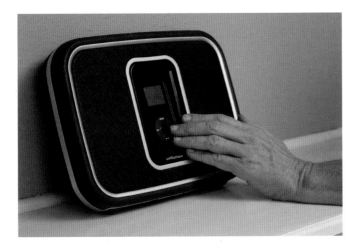

Some sink deeper into relaxation with calm, peaceful massage music while others find it distracting. Honor the wishes of the receiver. Soft, calming music that appeals to both the giver and receiver works best.

## CHECKLIST

1. Two clean soft towels or sheets.

2. Light blanket for warmth.

3. Pillow or bolster for underneath the legs.

4. Massage oil or lotion.

5. Tissues to wipe your hands.

6. Clock.

7. Water for the receiver during and after the massage.

8. Music.

9. Comfortable clothes.

# SELECTING THE SURFACE

## THE FLOOR

The floor is a massage surface that is available anywhere—at home, on vacation, and even outside. Be sure to place several cushions down to create a firm bed. You can use foam, a mattress pad, or a futon. Let the surface be soft and pliable.

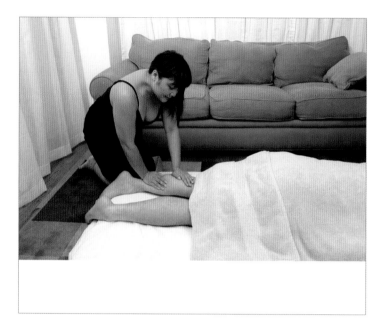

The floor offers plenty of room in all directions for both the giver and receiver to stretch out. Make sure you put some pillows under the receiver's knees while you are working on the front of the body.

The floor can be a challenge for the giver's body. Only massage for the length of time you are comfortable. If necessary take a few silent breaks during the massage to stretch. Your partner can relax and breathe.

## THE CHAIR

Using a chair works great for giving 15- or 20-minute rejuvenating rubs. The advantage of using a chair is that it is accessible to all of us and can be used anytime, anywhere. The chair is especially good for doing work on the back, but it rules out working on the entire body. It is not impossible to work on the other parts of the body using a chair, but it is a little difficult for the giver to remain comfortable.

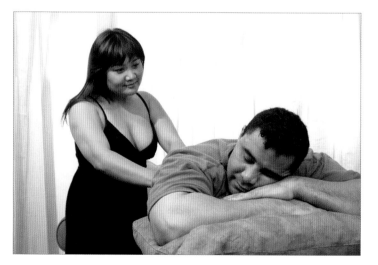

# THE TABLE

It is paramount that both the giver and the receiver are relaxed and comfortable during the massage. The floor or chair limits the duration that both the giver and receiver can maintain a feeling of comfort. A massage table makes it possible for both persons to be relaxed. It is designed to be ergonomically efficient for the giver. It can be adjusted so that a maximum amount of pressure can be applied with the least amount of effort. It allows the giver to be comfortable while moving around the table and using a wide variety of massage techniques.

The massage table works for just about anyone, whether adult or child. The giver can sit in a chair, a wheelchair, or even kneel on the table itself.

The softness of the massage table helps the receiver relax and let go. The headrest allows the receiver to rest his head comfortably in the horse-shoe shaped hole so that he can breathe easily throughout the entire massage.

A massage table is durable, comfortable, easily stored, and an invaluable addition to every home.

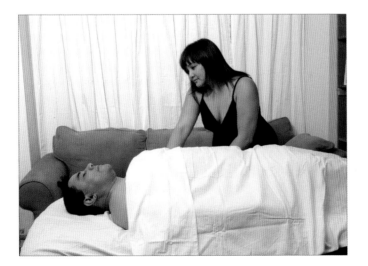

## A GOOD MASSAGE TABLE

A good massage table is a worthy investment. Today some massage tables are designed especially for the home. They are durable, affordable, and can be easily folded and put away when not in use. You can use your massage table at home, at a friend's house, or bring it on vacation.

## PROPER HEIGHT

Set the table height so that when you stand next to it, the top of your knuckles of your relaxed arms brush the table surface. This works for most people, however the proper height is the height that you find most comfortable. Always adjust the table to the height that works best for you.

## BEING COMFORTABLE

Being comfortable while you work is an important principle of Touch Communications Home Massage. The comfort of the giver resonates with the receiver and together they sink into a more relaxed state.

# THE GIVER AND THE RECEIVER

In Touch Communications Home Massage, the giver and the receiver are full participants in the healing process. The spirit of both persons is equally important. Massage is the willingness to share and communicate through the sense of touch. It is a two-way flow of energy—a conversation without words. This two-way mutual communication through the hands of the giver and the skin of the receiver is dependent upon both participants. It is a meditation for both partners, each engaging fully in the present moment of exchange.

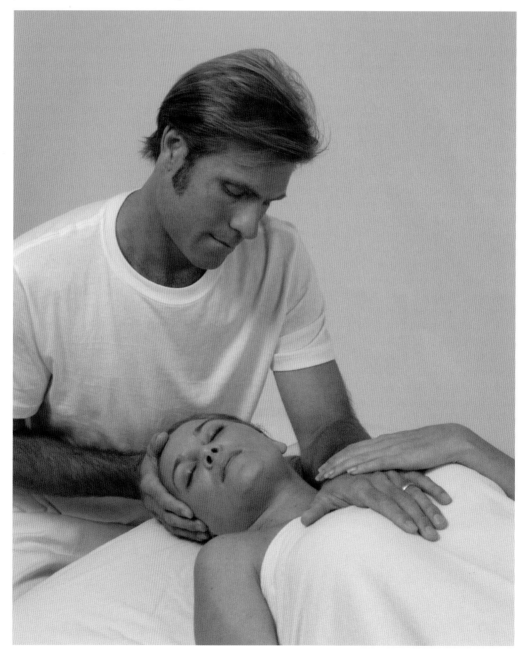

# THE GIVER

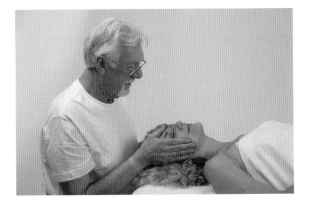

Massage is more about attitude than it is about talent and skill. When you give a massage, do it in a loving and joyful way. As giver, remind yourself of the three principles of Touch Communications Home Massage:

1. Create a safe space of honor and respect.

2. Encourage the art of massage by being present, being comfortable, having good intentions, and using your intuition.

3. Take the mystique out of massage techniques. Remember that techniques are important but for deep healing to occur, massage techniques must be blended with the art of massage.

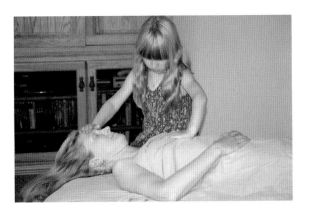

# THE RECEIVER

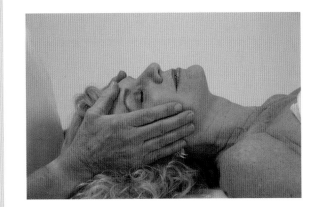

To benefit fully from a massage as the receiver, relax and let go of worries and concerns. As soon as you lie down, let yourself melt into the working surface. Close your eyes and become aware of your breathing and the parts of your body that move as you inhale and exhale. Rather than trying to help, surrender to the massage. Let the giver know if you particularly enjoy a certain stroke or movement.

Sounds are a wonderful way of releasing tension in your body. If the feeling arises, allow yourself the freedom to let go through deep breaths or "oohs" and "aahs." Let the giver know if you find the pressure too deep or too soft. If for any reason you feel uncomfortable or if you have to use the bathroom, let the giver know.

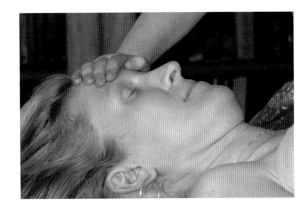

# TIPS FOR THE GIVER

Always wash your hands before giving a massage.

Remove all jewelry. Rings can scratch the skin and bracelets or necklaces can jingle, which causes a distraction. Rings or watches can also interfere with the free flow and natural movement of touching the receiver.

Wear loose clothing. Wear comfortable shoes or go barefoot.

Leave your daily worries and concerns behind and put a relaxed energy and focus into the massage.

Keep conversation to a minimum.

Remain present and be aware of the receiver's needs.

# TIPS FOR THE RECEIVER

Do not eat for about 90 minutes before the massage.

Remove all jewelry.

Remove make-up, contact lenses, and glasses.

The giver of the massage cannot "fix" anyone. Rather they assist or facilitate the healing process. To benefit from this process, the receiver must relax and be open to the touch of the giver.

During the massage, let the giver know if you want less or more pressure.

Remember, the massage is for your pleasure. Let the giver know your needs, whether you want music, the room is too cold, or you need a blanket for warmth.

# RELAX AND LET GO

Before giving a massage, take a few minutes to come down from your day's activities. You can meditate, listen to soft, soothing music, and take a few deep breaths.

During the massage, most of your attention will be on the receiver. It is important, however, to occasionally bring your attention back to yourself. Check to see that your breath is open, your shoulders are relaxed, and that you are not straining yourself in any way. Remember that touch is a highly sophisticated form of communication. If you are uncomfortable and stressed, that energy will be transmitted to the person on the table. If you are comfortable, relaxed, and calm, the receiver will feel the same. Stay in the full moment of the massage—no past and no future, just the beauty of your conversation through touch. If your thoughts drift away, gently bring them back to the moment by focusing on the skin beneath your hands.

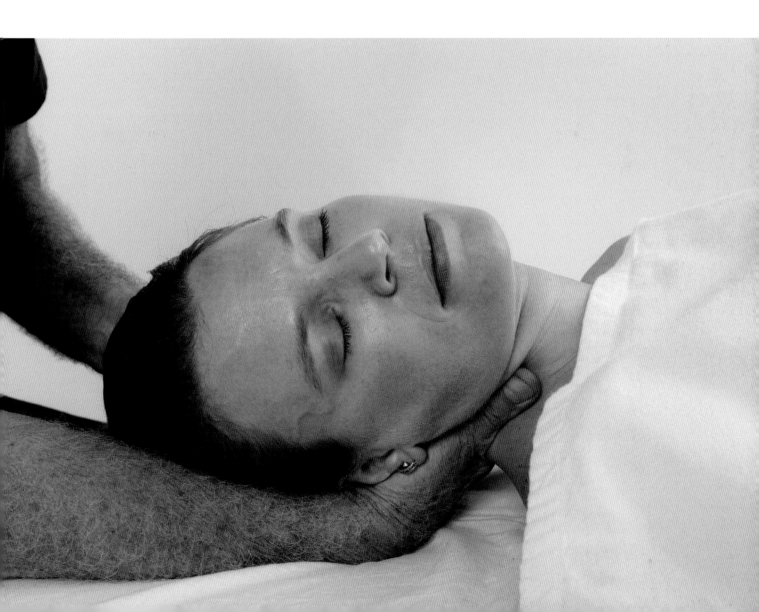

# CENTERING

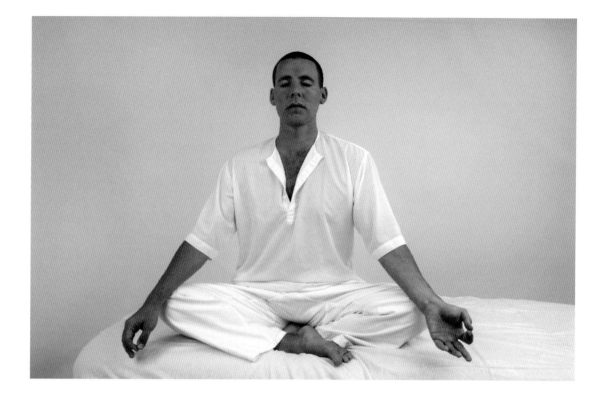

Before doing any kind of massage, you should spend a few minutes centering yourself. Emptying your mind allows your intuition, rather than your conscious mind, to guide the massage. This moves your energy down to the hara, just below the navel. This area, in Chinese and Japanese tradition, is considered the body's physical center of gravity and by extension the seat of one's spiritual energy.

Centering can be as simple as sitting quietly for a few minutes, or taking a deep breath and letting go of scattered thoughts while becoming aware of your body and breath. You can also take a few minutes and do a more formal type of exercise. These exercises can be done 10 to 30 minutes before the massage.

## CENTERING EXERCISE

This centering technique combines breath awareness with the phrase or mantra, "Let go." It is especially helpful when you are tense or fixating on a stressful situation or a negative thought or emotion.

Sit cross-legged or kneel down on the floor, putting a cushion under your buttocks. Do whatever it takes to make yourself comfortable. As you inhale, silently or out loud say, "Let." As you exhale, say "go" while letting go of all that is stressing you.

Repeat this exercise for three to five minutes.

# FOLLOWING YOUR INTUITION

A good "massager" is one who has the ability to combine input from his intuition and from their intellect as well. Balancing your knowledge of massage techniques with your intuition is vital to giving a healing massage.

Following the three principles of Touch Communications Home Massage—creating a safe place, encouraging the art of massage, and taking the mystique out of massage techniques—unleashes our innate ability to give an intuitive massage. In other words, it gives us confidence and opens the door to using our innate ability for healing touch. When we don't follow the principles—when we work under stress, are "in our ego," or try to prove our self-worth—we lose flexibility and openness. This also inhibits our ability to receive subtle information and clues from the receiver and from within ourselves. But when we focus on good intentions, promote comfort, become quiet and relaxed, we are able to listen and respond to the body of the receiver and sense her needs without saying a word.

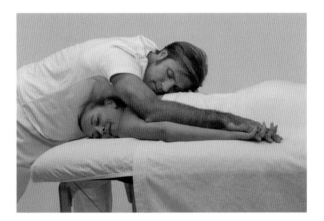

Honor the receiver. This means that you have the very best of intentions.

Take the mystique out of massage techniques. This means that you don't put all of your reliance into the massage techniques, but that you combine techniques with your innate ability of touch.

Apply the art of massage. This means that while you are giving a massage, you become quiet and comfortable in mind, body and spirit, returning you to your natural ability for healing touch.

# WHEN TO SAY NO

Massage is appropriate most of the time. It is non-invasive, relaxing, and generally considered a safe treatment for most people. However, there are times when massage is not advisable, when symptoms or a condition contraindicate its usage. Some of these deal with symptoms of disease. Some pertain to skin conditions. Others only apply to certain types of massage strokes or preclude working on a particular part of the body.

One contraindication that you should ALWAYS FOLLOW is a request from the receiver to stop what you are doing or to not work on a specific area. Just acknowledge the request without judgement or questions. If you are following the First Principle of "Creating a safe place of honor and respect" (page 54), this will come naturally.

A good rule to follow: when you are in doubt, check with your physician.

## TOTAL CONTRAINDICATIONS

Contagious diseases or infections including colds or flu
Recent operations or acute injuries
Skin disease
Fever

## LOCAL AREAS TO AVOID

Varicose veins
Bruises
Cuts and abrasions
Undiagnosed pain
Swollen areas and areas of inflammation

## MEDICAL CONDITIONS

Cancer, diabetes, heart problems, osteoperosis and other bone disease,
and other medical conditions do not mean that massage cannot take place.
With these and other conditions, it is best to check with your physician.

The very young, the elderly and pregnant women all should be
handled with great care. Please refer to pages 147, 184 and 189
as well as the Suggested Reading section at the end of this book
for more information.

# TIME TO TALK

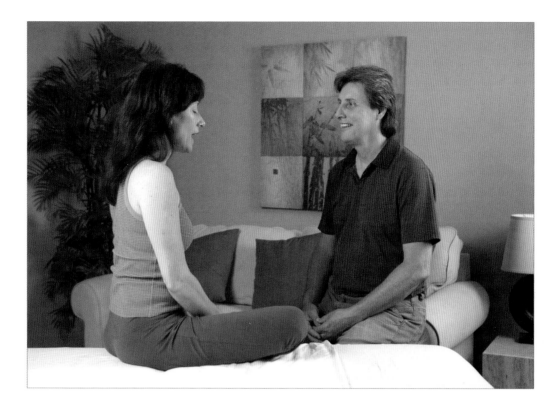

Before you start the massage, spend a few minutes discussing your partner's needs. Listen to any concerns. If this is the first time massaging the person, ask if she has any places on the body that you should avoid massaging.

Check on the time available for the massage. It helps to have some idea of the amount of time you will be massaging the receiver. Ask if she would like soft music or she would prefer quiet.

Massage involves intimate touch, so it is very important to eliminate any concerns. Make your conversation brief but complete so the massage can occur without interruptions. A few minutes of mutual understanding will alleviate any worries for both the giver and receiver.

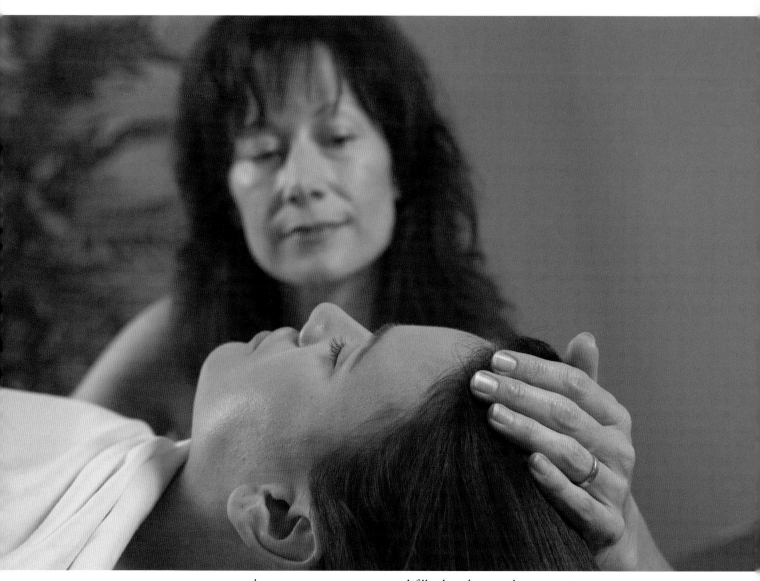

When we are present and filled with good
intentions, our healing hands communicate love and
compassion to the receiver.

# KEEPING YOUR HANDS SOFT

Many students of massage, as well as many professional massage therapists, have a difficult time accepting that their hands can be soft—that is, free from tension, while still applying enough pressure. Hence, they resist the notion of keeping their hands soft. They work with tension in their hands and then wonder why they are not able to feel and sense the subtle differences in the tissue.

Using our relaxed body to apply pressure while keeping our hands soft not only feels better to the receiver, it indicates to the giver how deep to go, where to spend more time, and how fast or how slow to move our hands.

Becoming quiet and improving our awareness of our body is vital to releasing our accumulated stress. Without awareness, we live in the illusion that everything is fine, and that it is normal to feel tense and uptight.

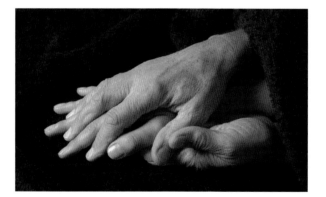

We can practice releasing the tension in our hands at any time, including while we are giving a massage. Try this exercise:

With your hands soft, center your attention to different parts of your hands, continue to release the tension out of your hands. Once you have done that bring your attention back to where you started and again relax your hands and let go of all tension.

We do not release tension from our hands or from any other part of our body in one big swoop, but rather in tiny increments.

# OILS AND LOTIONS

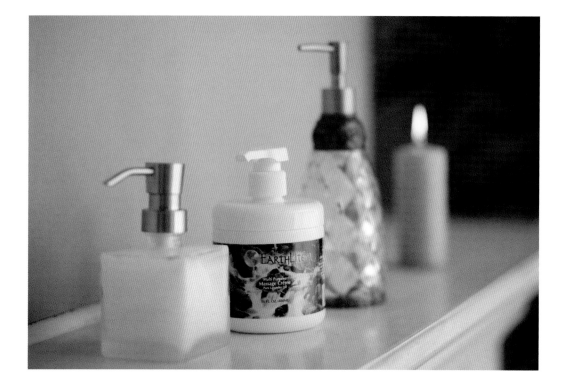

Using a lubricant when massaging helps your hands glide easily while still creating the necessary friction to be effective. Whether you use a massage lotion or oil is a matter of preference. However, it is best to use pure products formulated from all natural ingredients.

Massage oils are applied easily to the skin for a light, even glide and smooth workability. Pure cold-pressed oils are ideal for therapists looking for natural products.

Pure almond oil is an excellent emollient (softening and soothing to the skin) and also helps the skin to balance its loss of moisture. The aroma is light, slightly sweet, and nutty.

Massage lotions are a combination of oil and cream. They are the preference of many massage therapists. Lotions create a smooth friction that allows for deeper work. Lotions don't absorb as quickly into the skin. Massage lotions can be purchased in bath and body shops, health food stores, and in massage supply stores.

# APPLYING THE OIL OR LOTION

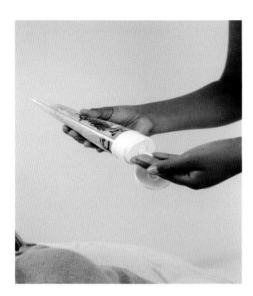

First, apply the lubricant to your hands and rub it on. If the lubricant feels cold, rub it into your hands until it feels warm enough to apply. Using a gliding stroke, cover the part of the body you want to work on first.

Be sparing with the amount of lubricant you apply. Use enough to glide along the tissue while still maintaining a gentle friction. Using too much lubricant makes the body too slippery and difficult to work on. If you apply too much, do not wipe it off. Instead, softly pat the lubricated area with a towel to remove the excess.

Keep the lubricant dispenser on or near you. Do not place it on the massage table near enough to the receiver where they might brush against it. Leave the bottle open so you don't have to pause to open or close the lid.

It is a nice touch to have a bowl with hot water in the room in which to place the lotion. This warms the lotion and guards against an abrupt sensation of cold to the receiver.

Never apply the oil or lotion directly onto the receiver. Apply it to your hands, then spread it where you want to work

If you have both massage lotion and oil in the room, give the receiver the option of choosing which he would prefer.

Always check with your partner to see if he or she has any known allergy or skin conditions. When possible, use a hypoallergenic product.

# DRAPING

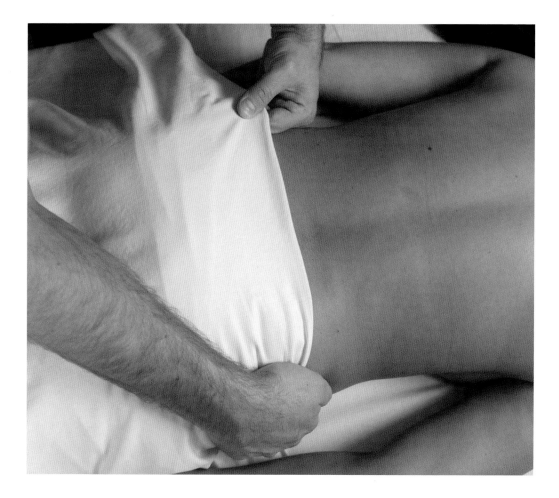

Draping plays an essential role in creating a secure environment for the receiver to feel safe and honored. Make sure you convey to the receiver that you respect her privacy and vulnerability and that you appreciate her trust.

There are many different stages of undress, from being completely naked under the covers to wearing underwear or articles of clothing during the massage. If this is someone's first time receiving a massage, you may have to inform her of the options and then explain that the decision is strictly up to her.

Everything you do during a massage, including draping, should be done with a great sense of care and deliberation to make the receiver feel relaxed and secure.

A flat twin-sized sheet provides a very effective, secure cover. Uncover only the part of the body you are massaging. The sheet should protect the rest of the body. For comfort, some people prefer their arms or feet to be outside of the covers. Ask your partner what feels most comfortable to them.

Sometimes people need assistance getting on and off the table. This might also involve your assistance with the draping, and may necessitate turning your head away while holding the covering material. Remember, if you approach draping from a place of honor and respect, you will create a space of security and trust and you will be able to handle any situation comfortably.

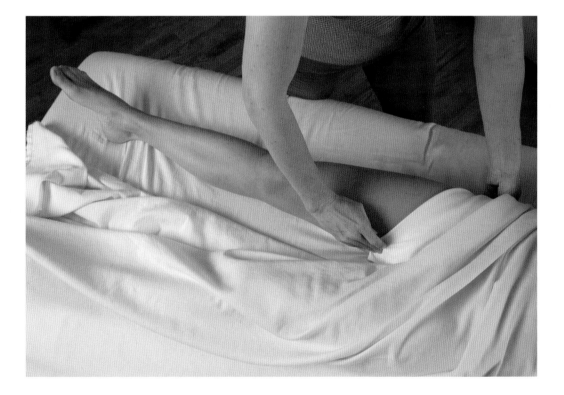

# PROPER BODY STANCE

Using good body mechanics and leaning into the movements improves efficiency, power, and strength while reducing stress on the giver. Use your body to apply pressure and keep your hands soft. Pay attention to your own body and mind while you are giving a massage.

The following stances are merely a guideline for you to follow. Use whatever method you feel comfortable in and relax your stance. Breathing is one of the best ways to relax your body.

## THE HORSE STANCE

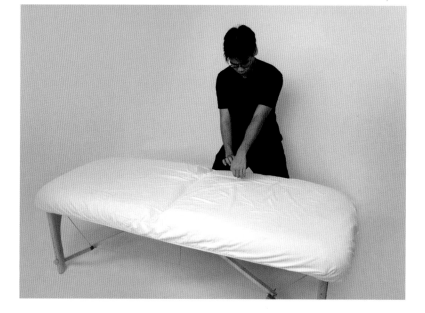

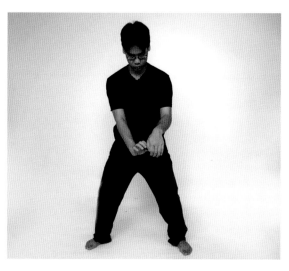

In the horse stance, both feet are pointed into the table. The knees are slightly flexed and the back remains erect and relaxed. The horse stance involves shifting your weight from side to side.

Pay attention to your shoulders, hands, and legs while working. If you feel tension in your body, move around and find a way to get comfortable.

# THE ARCHER STANCE

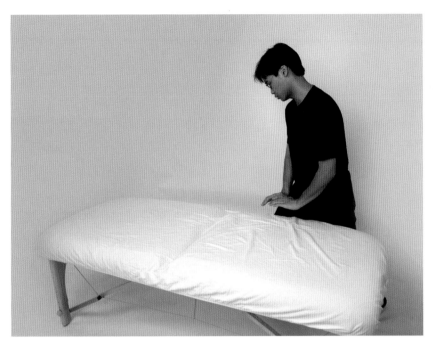

The archer stance is the most commonly used position. For the archer stance, the feet are positioned so that an imaginary line drawn through the center of one foot at the arch passes through the other foot at mid-heel. This foot position provides a solid, stable foundation for the giver to lean into or pull back on a massage stroke. By shifting weight from one foot to the other, the giver can perform long, rhythmic strokes. Breathe, relax, and use your body. Keep your hands soft.

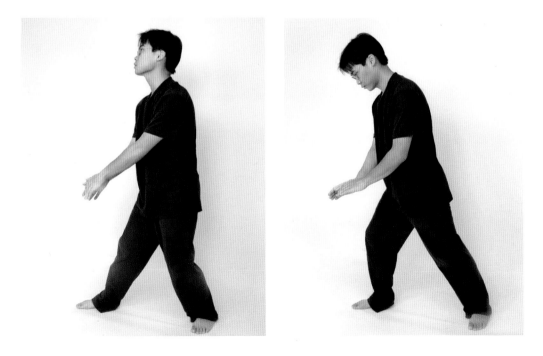

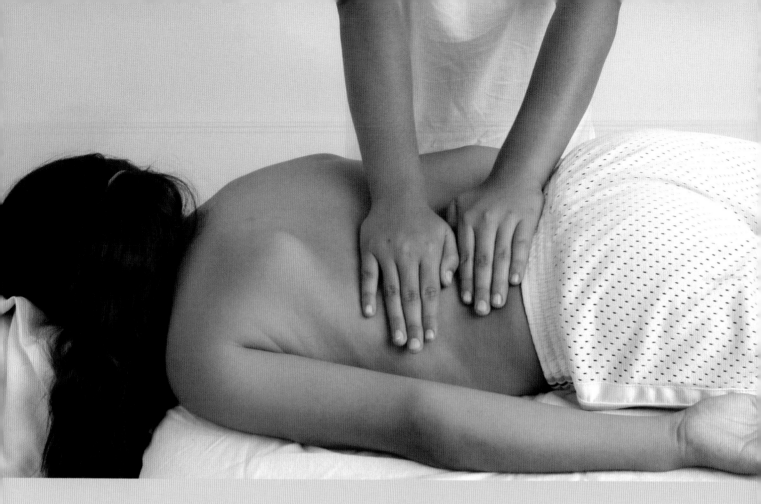

## CHAPTER SIX

# SIMPLE STROKES

Your hands are perfectly designed
for giving a massage

Most massage treatments are a combination of massage strokes. These essential strokes provide you with the basic movements needed to perform a full-body massage. Although the rhythmic, flowing movements of these individual strokes form the basic components of massage, there are many more variations of strokes.

Slower movements are generally soothing and relaxing, while faster movements tend to energize and invigorate. For home massage treatment, we recommend that you work slowly and deliberately, using your relaxed body to apply pressure while keeping your hands soft. As you become more comfortable and confident, experiment by creating your own movements and routines.

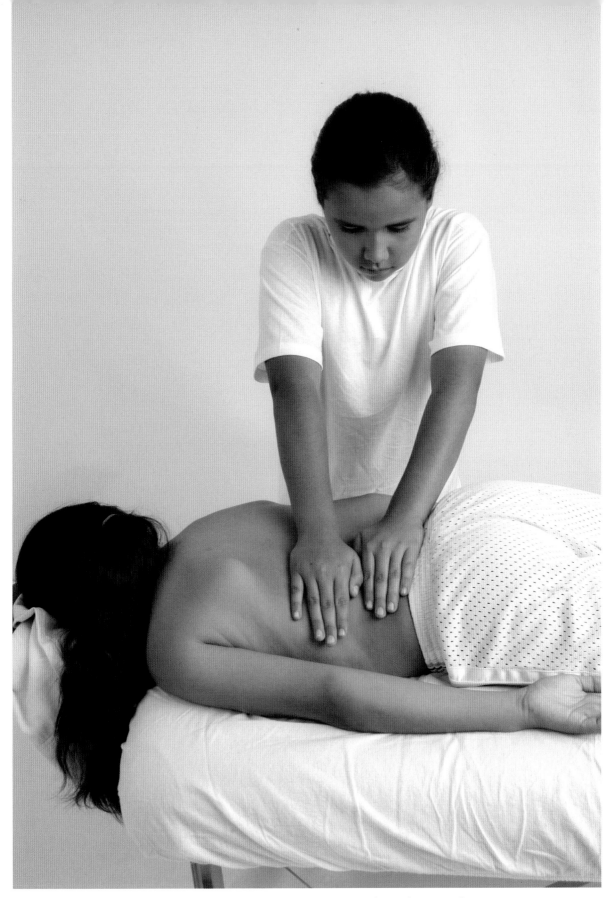

Practice these strokes with a light heart. You don't have to hit every note perfectly to give a good massage.

# GENTLE STROKE

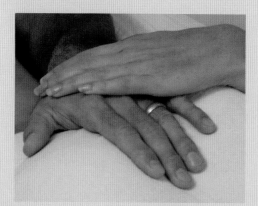

Gentle touch. It is amazing how much so little will do!

Gentle touch means simply laying your hands on your partner's covered body without movement. Let your hands rest in a peaceful position. You can lay your gentle touch on your partner's back, abdomen, heart, feet, and head. Breathe slowly and, when possible, synchronize your breathing with the inhale and exhale of your partner's breathing. Become as comfortable and present as possible. Your willingness to be still, to do nothing, and to expect nothing promotes a sense of calm and peace within the receiver.

This gentle touch without movement should always be used to initiate the massage. It signals your partner that the massage is about to begin, creates a necessary connection and sets the tone for a continual sense of safety, comfort, and relaxation. Guided by your own intuition, this stroke can be used at any time during the massage. It is also a gentle way to end the massage.

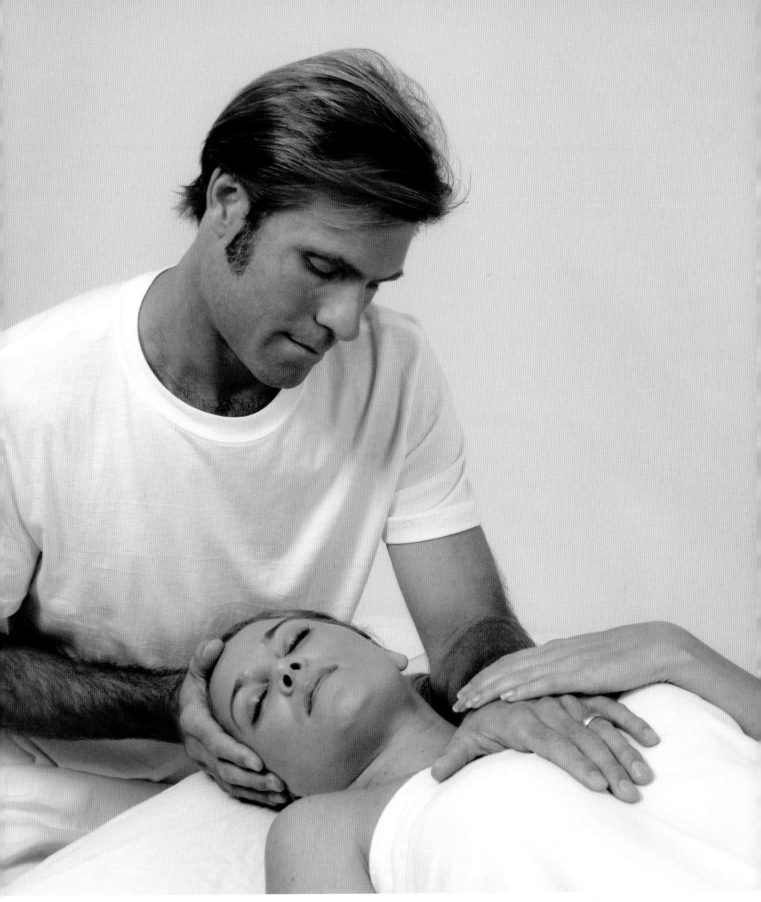

This soft gentle touch without movement feels deeply relaxing and comforting to both the giver and the receiver.

# EFFLEURAGE STROKE

## Gliding Stroke

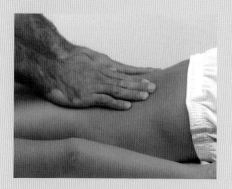

Lay your relaxed hands onto your partner with full contact
and your fingers softly together.

For your own safety and protection and for that of any family member or
friend, please take a moment to review the Contraindications (page 78)
prior to practicing the strokes and techniques.

After the application of the gentle touch used to initiate the massage, the effleurage
stroke is often next in sequence. The simple name for the effleurage stroke is the
gliding stroke. This stroke is the easiest massage movement to learn and one of the
most used during the massage. It is excellent for spreading lubricant on the skin. The
effleurage stroke is applied using hands, fingers, or your forearm in a succession of
light or deep gliding motions. It is the most versatile stroke. When the gliding stroke is
applied with more pressure, it can produce increased circulation of blood and lymph
fluids and can reduce muscle spasms and tension.

The simplicity and ease of applying this movement, particularly when done in a rhythmic fashion, makes this an effective manipulation to use repetitively while gradually
increasing the pressure. It is also excellent for warming up an area to prepare for
more detailed work. The effleurage stroke is the best stroke to use when working
over sensitive areas, such as the abdomen.

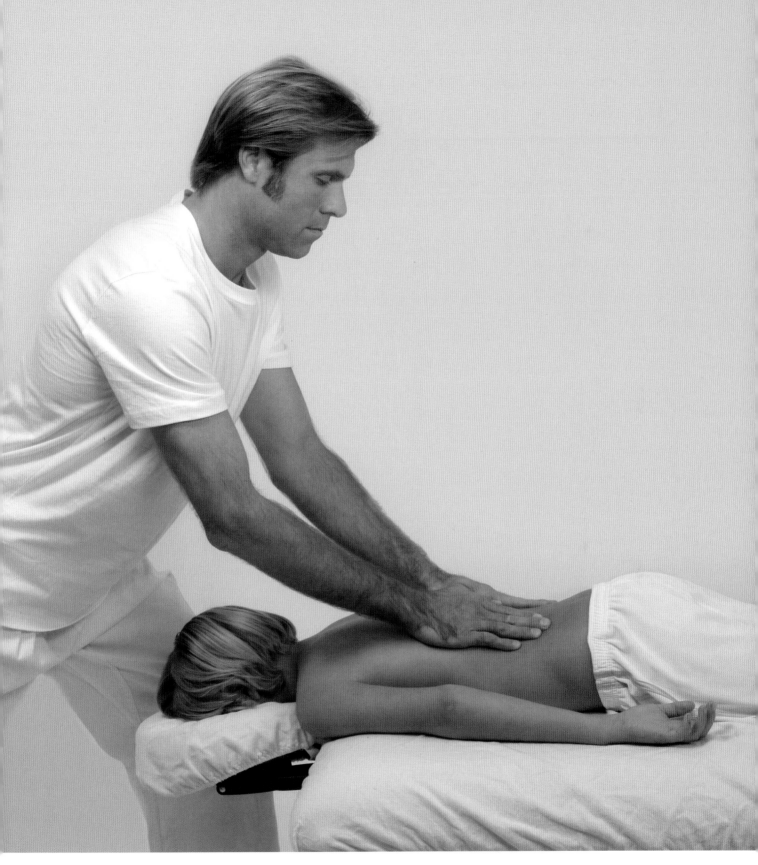

The back provides an excellent canvas to practice the gliding stroke with your partner. Be present and pay attention to the sensation of the tissue beneath your hands.

# PETRISSAGE STROKE
## Kneading Stroke

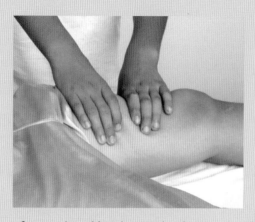

Move forward and back in a rhythmic way when
doing the petrissage stroke.

The petrissage stroke is best to use after you have warmed the tissue with the gliding
stroke. Petrissage movements include the wringing, lifting, and rolling of tissue and skin.
To prevent pinching, the kneading stroke should be done slowly and with soft hands.
If the tissue is lifted and squeezed too tightly or too rapidly, it will be uncomfortable
for your partner.

The kneading stroke can be used to soothe tired, aching and overworked muscles.
The petrissage movements can stimulate the skin, improve muscle tone, encourage
the elimination of waste products from tissues, and help break down scar tissue.
When done correctly with a smooth rhythm, kneading is one of the most pleasurable
strokes to receive.

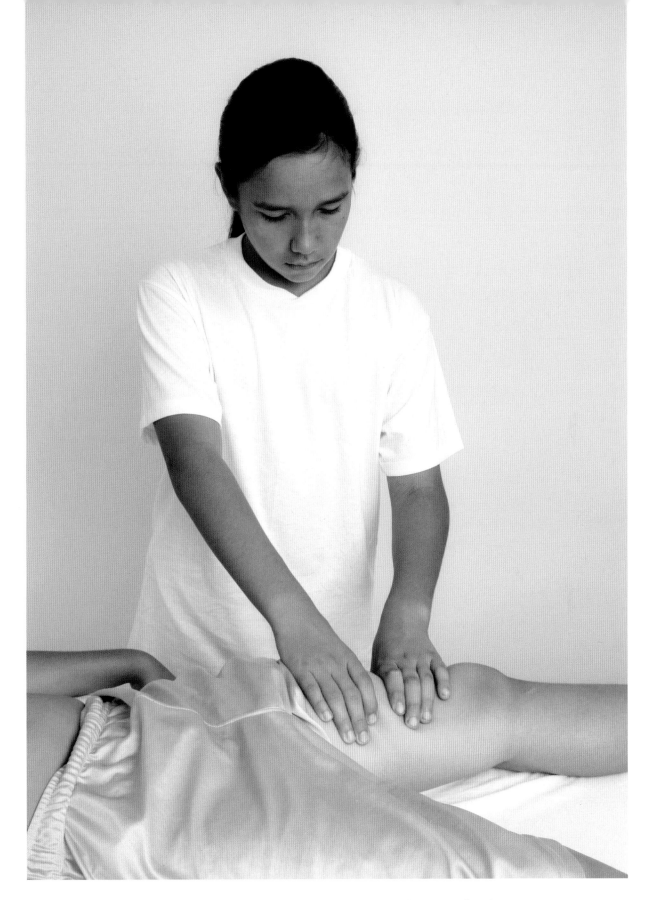

Let all thoughts leave your mind, relax your body,
make full contact with soft hands, and enjoy the rhythm.

# THUMB CIRCLING STROKE

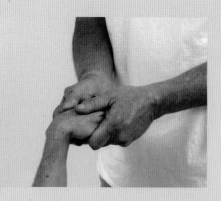

*Thumb circling is good for loosening deep, chronic muscle tension.*

Thumb circling can be applied gently on places like the forehead. It can be a penetrating stroke over areas such as the lower back, between the shoulder blades and the spine, and on the calf muscles. Be sure to warm the area before using thumb circling, especially before doing deep work.

Place the pads of your thumbs on the area you are working and gradually lean into the flesh. Next, make small, penetrating circular movements. It is best to keep your hands and thumbs soft when doing this move. Tightening your hands and thumbs will not feel good to the receiver and may cause your thumbs and hands to become sore and irritated. Only apply as much pressure as is comfortable for you and the receiver.

If you are uncomfortable using your thumbs, you can use a knuckling circular motion to achieve the same effect. Sometimes the pads of your fingers are used for this stroke. Once again, lean into the move and keep your hands soft.

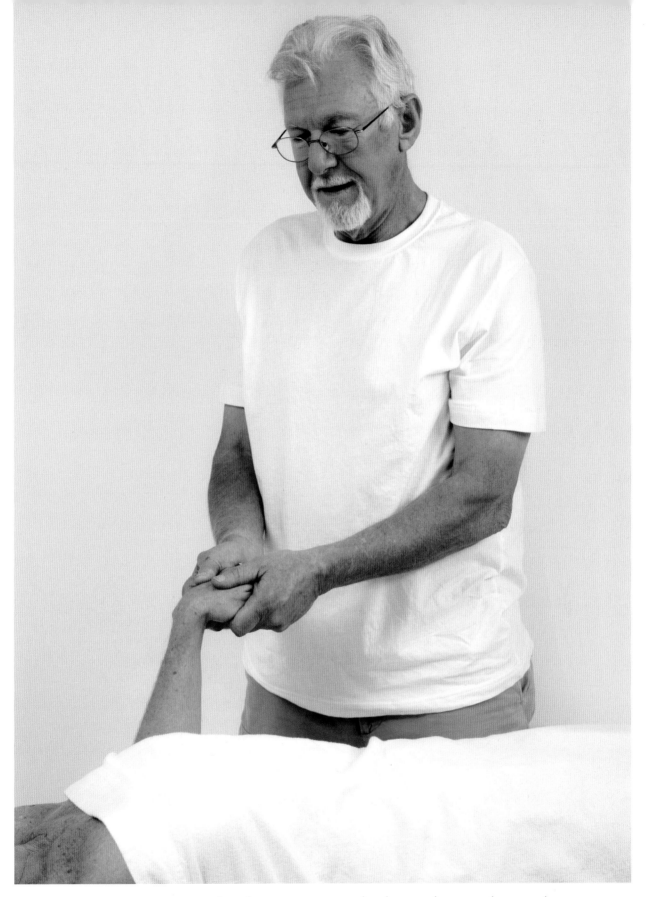

You can use your thumbs one at a time, both together, or alternately, depending on the area you are massaging.

# COMPRESSION

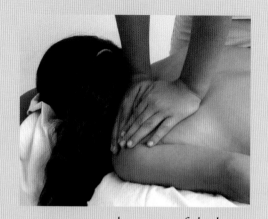

The compression stroke is one of the best to use
through clothing or through the drape.

Compression strokes are simple and do just that: compress. There are variations on this stroke, all of which are applied in a similar manner — by compressing the tissue, holding for a moment, then slowly releasing. This stroke slows the blood flow for a moment, then allows the blood to flush through the area, increasing circulation, delivering needed nutrients, and removing toxins.

The heel of the hand can be used to compress the back of the leg, the lower back, or the shoulders. Whole hands can be wrapped around an arm or foot to squeeze and compress. Fingertips can be placed on the temples or the jaw to lightly compress, hold, and release.

When using the heels of the hands, slowly add pressure by leaning your body into your hands, hold for a moment, then slowly release by moving your body back. As with the other strokes, apply the compression stroke rhythmically. The body likes rhythm. It is a comforting movement, similar to a rocking baby.

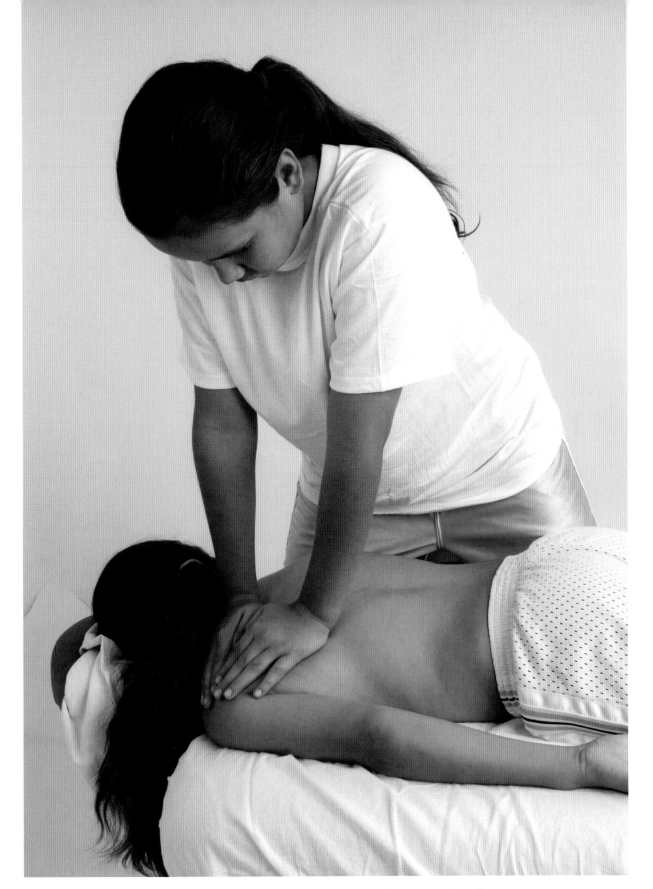

The compression stroke is especially good for boosting local circulation, clearing toxins and lymph, and reducing tension in the area you are working.

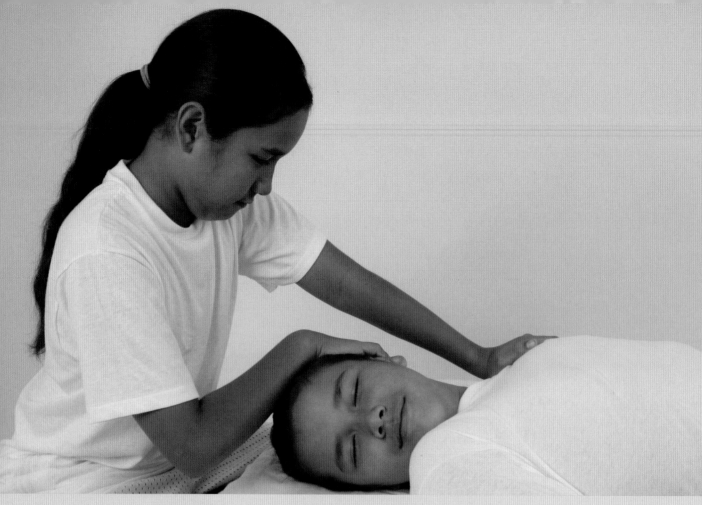

## CHAPTER SEVEN

# MASSAGE ROUTINES

Now that you are familiar with massage strokes, it's time to move on to massage routines. If massage strokes are the notes, then massage routines are putting the notes together into a song.

Massage routines are specific strokes linked in a variety of ways to various parts of the body. Massage routines can be performed on a particular part of the body such as the back or arm, or they can be combined to form a wonderful full-body massage. A massage routine can be a planned sequence of strokes or intuitive from the beginning to the end of the massage. A good idea is to develop a massage routine but always improvise your moves to meet the needs and wants of your partner.

# ONE POSSIBLE SEQUENCE

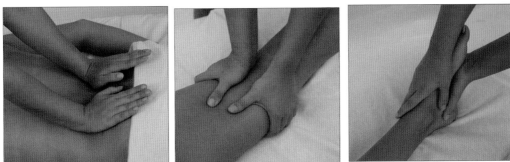

The Back and
Shoulders

The Legs

The Feet

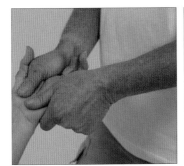

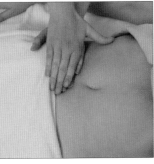

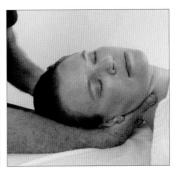

The Arms and Hands

The Abdomen

The Head and Neck

NOTE: Please take a moment to refer to the Contraindications (page 78)
before beginning the massage routine.

A good way to begin your massage is with strokes that relax and warm your partner's muscles. These are usually the long, sweeping effleurage strokes. After your partner is relaxed and his muscles have been warmed, you can apply more specific and deeper techniques. As an example, if your partner is a runner, then you may want to spend more time doing thumb circling to the legs. If your partner indicates that a certain stroke or a particular part of his body you are working on feels especially good, then spend more time there.

A good rule to follow is to transition one stroke smoothly into the next, the same way an accomplished dancer flows from one move into another. At first combining these strokes may seem a bit awkward but, with a little practice, you will forget about the notes and experience the melody, rhythm and song.

# THE BACK AND SHOULDERS

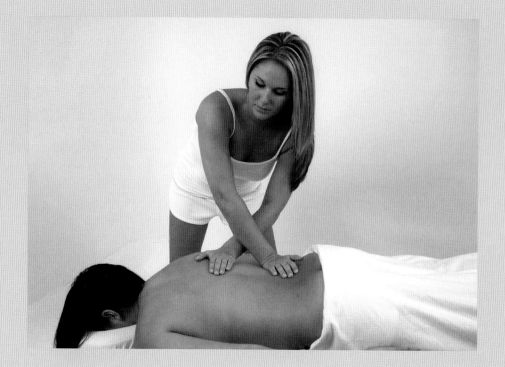

After applying the initiating gentle touch, the back provides a wonderful starting point for your massage journey. It is the part of the body that most people are comfortable touching and the part of the body where most people are comfortable being touched. It is the largest part of the body to work and the easiest on which to practice those long gliding strokes.

There are many nerves branching out from the spine to all parts of the body. A good back massage can have a calming effect on your entire nervous system. Slow, smooth, rhythmic strokes relax, while fast strokes invigorate. For family massage, we recommend that you use these slower movements. They assist in removing the stresses of our daily lives and create a general sense of well-being.

## PALM COMPRESSION STROKE
### Lower Back

**1** Place the palms of your hands on the sacrum (the flat, bony area at the base of the spine). Slowly lean forward while keeping your arms straight. This move stretches and opens the lower back. Continue to lean forward and hold for about five seconds. Maintain contact with the palms of your hands as you slowly lean backwards to release the pressure.

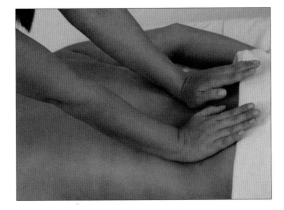

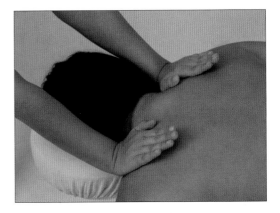

**2** Next, move your hands so they are about two to three inches apart, then repeat this entire stroke several times. Remember to lean in slowly, hold without movement for five seconds, and maintain contact as you slowly release.

**3** After completing the lower back, place your hands on the shoulders and apply the compression stroke. Lean in, hold for five seconds, and maintain contact as your slowly release.

# EFFLEURAGE STROKE
## Back and Shoulders

This long, gliding effleurage stroke covers the entire back. It is a good stroke to initiate and to complete the work on the back. It also warms the muscles for detailed work.

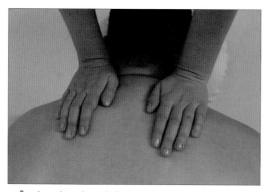

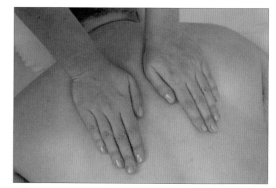

1 Apply the lubricant to your hands. Place your hands on either side of the spine with your fingers pointing towards the feet. Leave space between your thumbs for the spine.

2 Using the flat of your relaxed hands lean forward into your hands and glide all the way down to the sacrum.

3 Once you have reached the sacrum, draw your hands back up to the top of the shoulders.

4 Next, circle your hands around the shoulders, molding them to the contour of the shoulders. Complete this stroke by returning to the original starting point. You can repeat this stroke several times.

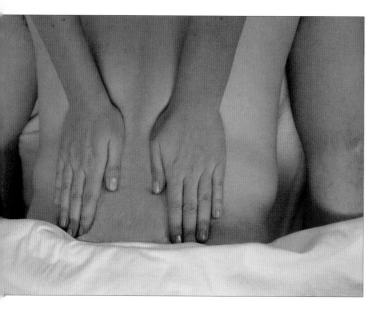

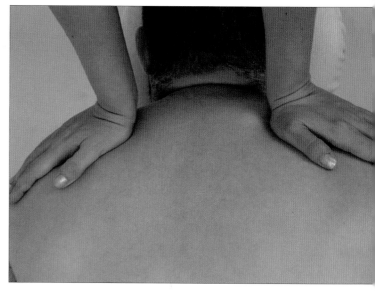

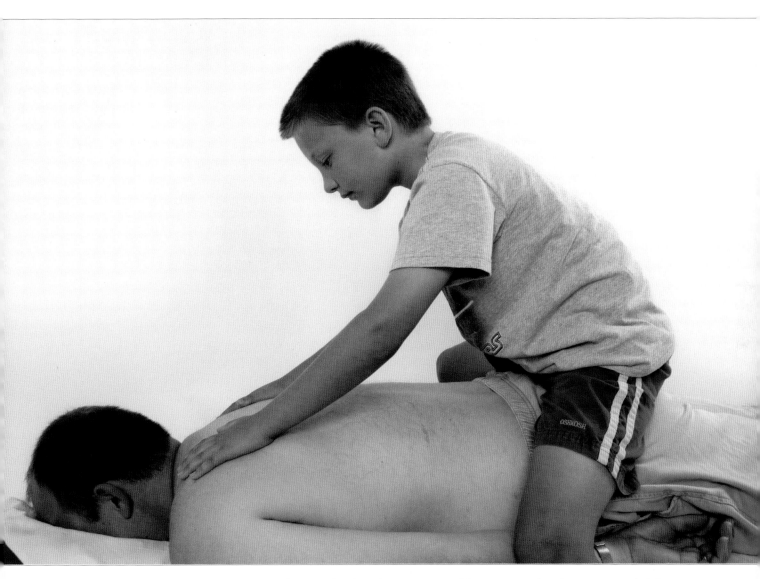

The gliding effleurage stroke on the back is a very effective stroke for young children
to do while sitting on the receiver, gliding their hands up the spine
from the lower back to the shoulders and down again.

## EFFLEURAGE STROKE
### Lower Back

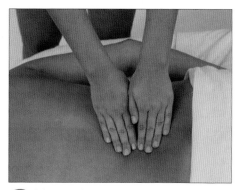

**2** Next, slowly move away from the spine down to the waist. It is important when doing this stroke to move slowly and stay present.

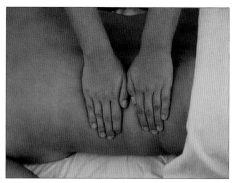

**3** Complete this stroke by grasping the flesh with soft open hands and leaning back. This is a sensitive part of the body. Too much pressure will feel uncomfortable and too little will feel like a tickle.

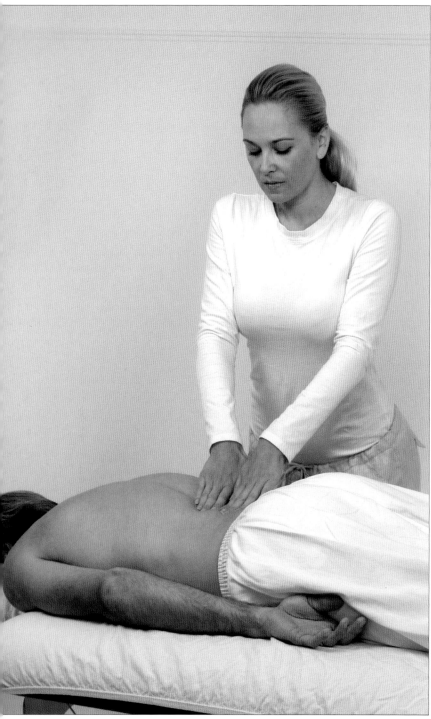

**1** For this stroke you are working on the side opposite from where you are standing. Place the pads of your fingers against the far side of the lower spine.

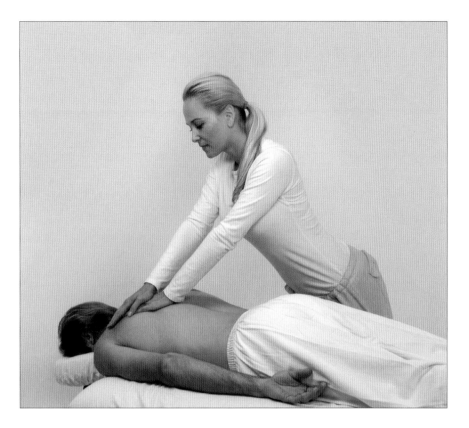

# HAND ON HAND PETRISSAGE STROKE
## Shoulder and Scapula

1 For this stroke, you will be standing on one side of your partner and facing the head of the table. Next, reach across your partner to the opposite shoulder. With your hands conforming to the body, put one hand on top of the other and place them on the shoulder.

2 Start with the muscle between the neck and the shoulders. Use both hands to grasp the flesh, lean back and lift the muscle. Maintain contact as you stroke in a circular motion.

3 Conform your hands to the body as its shape changes. Continue to circle around with both hands in a smooth, rhythmic way. Repeat this stroke on the other side.

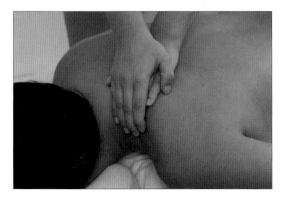

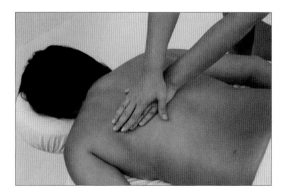

## DETAILED EFFLEURAGE STROKE
### Between Spine and Shoulder Blade

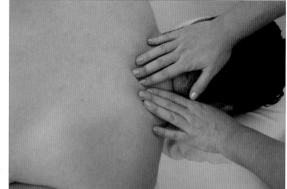

Use your finger pads to apply the gliding (effleurage) stroke between the spine and the shoulder blade. Start at the top of the back between the spine and the shoulder blade and massage to the end of the shoulder blade. That is approximately at the end of the crease of the armpit.

## THUMB CIRCLING STROKE
### Between Spine and Shoulder Blade

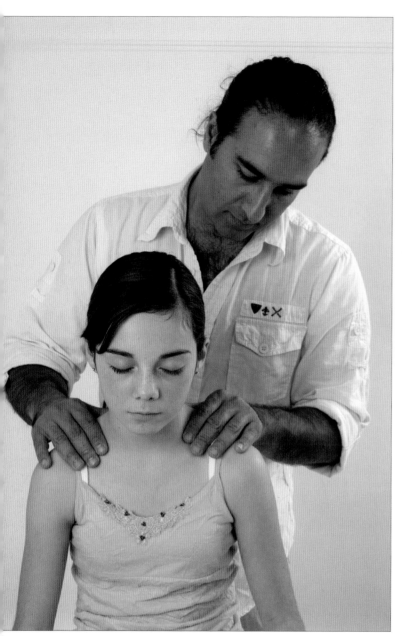

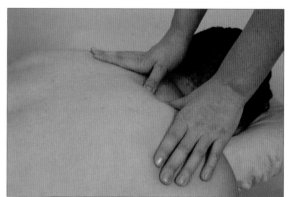

Continue to work this area by making thumb circles between the shoulder blade (scapula) and the spine. Your movements should be slow and rhythmic. Use your body to lean into the stroke. Remember to use the pads of your thumbs as opposed to using the tips of your thumbs.

Throughout the massage, keep most of your attention on your partner and some of it on yourself. While working on your partner's shoulders or any other part of her body, make sure that your hands are soft, that you are comfortable, and that your breath is open.

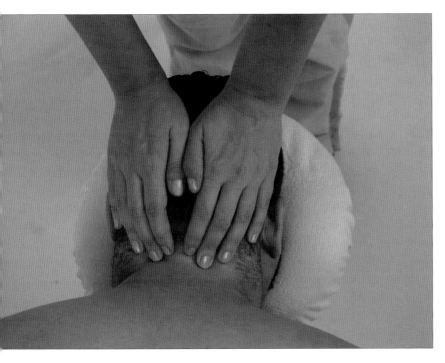

## FINGER CIRCLING STROKE
### Groove Between the Head and Neck

Standing at the head of the table, place your finger pads in the groove between the head and the neck. This groove is called the occipital ridge. Make circles with the pads of your fingers. It is best when these circles are done slowly with firm pressure.

This stroke is excellent for relieving stress in the head and neck.

## COMPRESSION STROKE
### Back

Place one hand on the sacrum and the other hand on the upper back. Lean in with your body, hold for approximately five seconds, then release pressure slowly while maintaining contact with your partner. You can repeat this stroke several times.

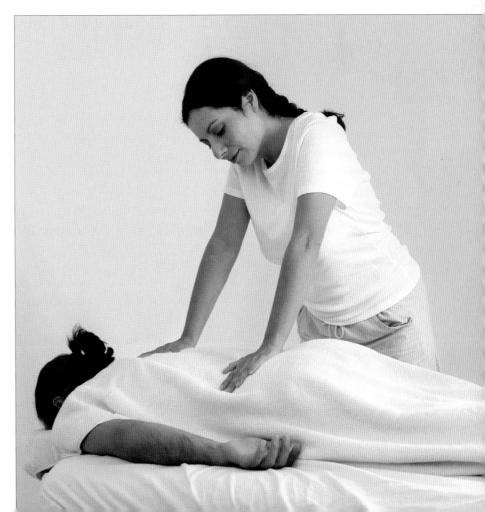

# THE LEGS

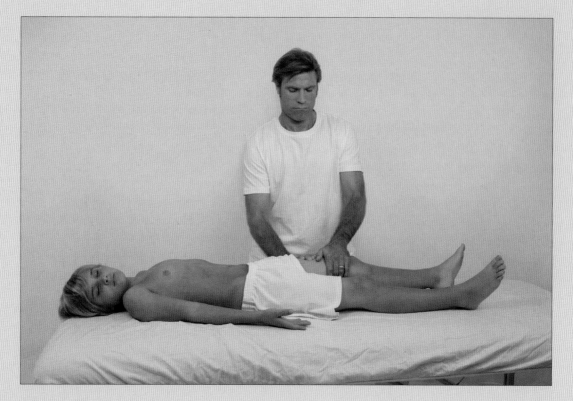

Aches and pains in our back and neck are often caused by tight muscles in the legs. Whether one leads a highly active or a more sedentary life, everyone can greatly benefit from a leg massage.

A good leg massage will circulate the blood and lymphatic system, loosen tight muscles, and leave the receiver feeling invigorated. You can apply deep pressure over the thicker areas on the leg, but be especially careful when working over the back of the knee. Only apply a very light pressure when working over the knee and bony areas of the leg.

If your partner has varicose veins, avoid them entirely and use a light pressure over the rest of the leg.

# EFFLEURAGE STROKE
## Back of Legs

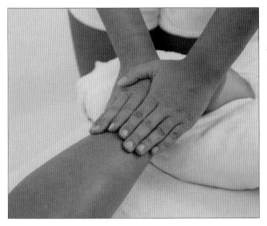

**1** For this stroke, you are in the archer stance. The effleurage stroke is used to initiate and complete a leg massage. Start at the ankle, with both hands soft. Remember, this is a gliding stroke.

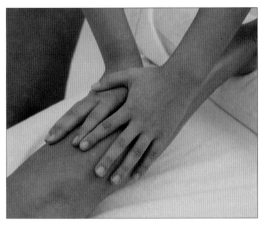

**2** Lean into your hands to apply even, firm pressure up the calf muscle. Glide over the back of the knee with a light touch. If your partner has varicose veins, avoid working directly on them.

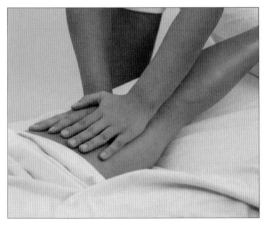

**3** Once you get past the knee and into the fleshy area of the thigh, you can increase the pressure. From the thigh, bring both of your hands to the outside of the leg and drag them back to the ankle. Repeat this move several times. Each time you stroke up the leg, stroke up at a different angle so you eventually cover or "paint" the entire leg.

# PETRISSAGE STROKE
## Back of Legs

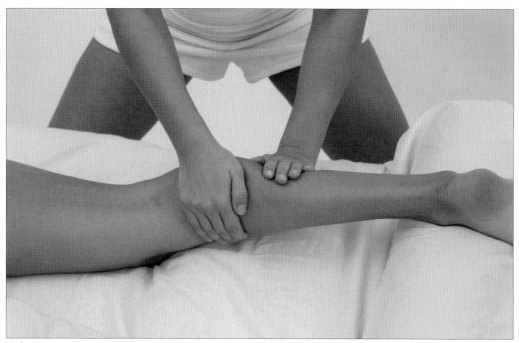

**1** Use the horse stance for this stroke. You may notice that your body sways with this stroke. Begin with the lower leg. Place one hand on the outside of the leg, with the heel of that hand touching the table. Place your other hand on the inside of the leg, with your fingertips touching the table.

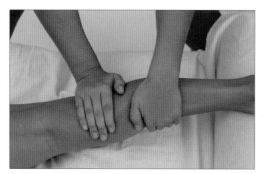

**2** Next, take hold of a large portion of flesh and pull your hands up the sides, changing hand positions. Continue to lift the tissue, gradually working over the entire calf muscle. Your intention with this stroke is to lift the muscle off of the bone. Use full, firm soft hands.

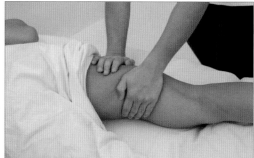

**3** When you have completed the petrissage stroke on the lower part of the leg, move to the upper part of the leg and do the same stroke on the thigh. Take hold of a large portion of flesh because too little may feel like a pinch. Keep kneading until the thigh muscles feel warm and relaxed.

# THUMB CIRCLING STROKE
## Back of Legs

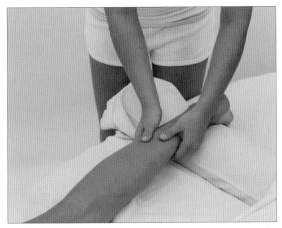

**1** Place your thumbs just below the calf muscle on both sides of the leg.

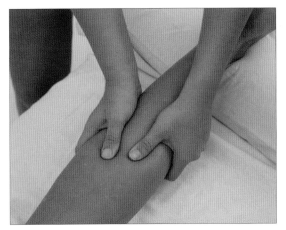

**2** Begin thumb circling and gradually move up the back of the calf muscle. Remember to stay away from the area behind the knee.

**3** Keeping your hands and thumbs soft, lean into them and continue circling up the thigh. To return, glide your hands down the leg to the ankle and begin again. Repeat this move several times.

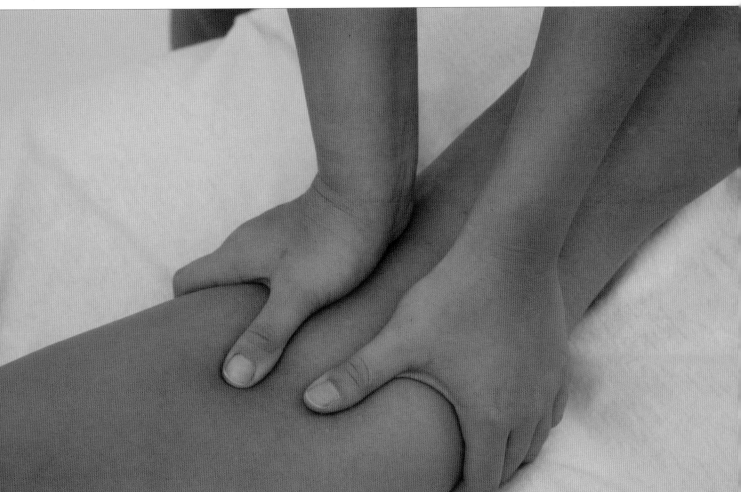

# EFFLEURAGE STROKE
## Front of Leg

**1** For your comfort, the archer stance is best for this stroke. Start at the ankle, with the hands on either side of the leg.

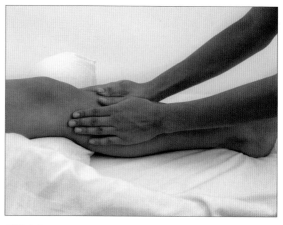

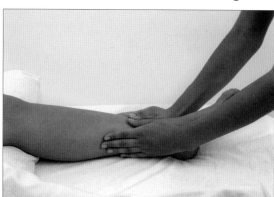

**2** Next, gently lean into your hands and glide up the sides of the calf muscle.

**3** Stroke (with no pressure) over the knee. When beyond the knee, increase the pressure and continue up the thigh. Be sensitive about your partner's privacy as you work the inner thigh. To return, bring your hands to the outside of the leg and drag them back to the ankle. You can repeat this stroke several times.

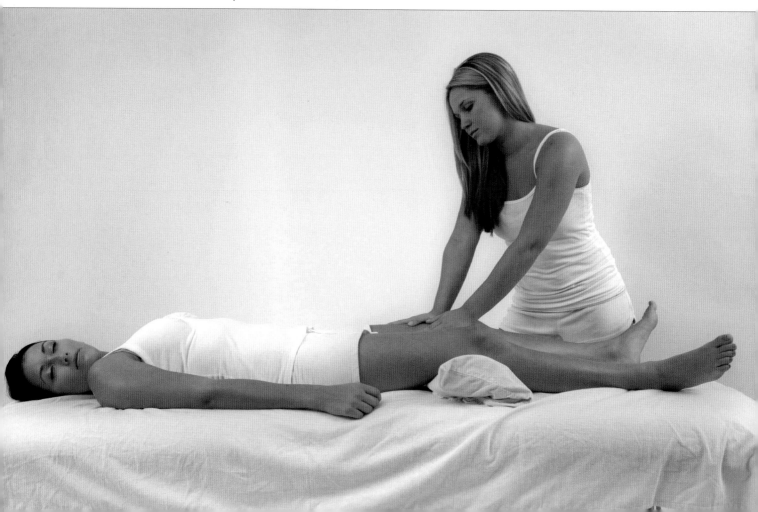

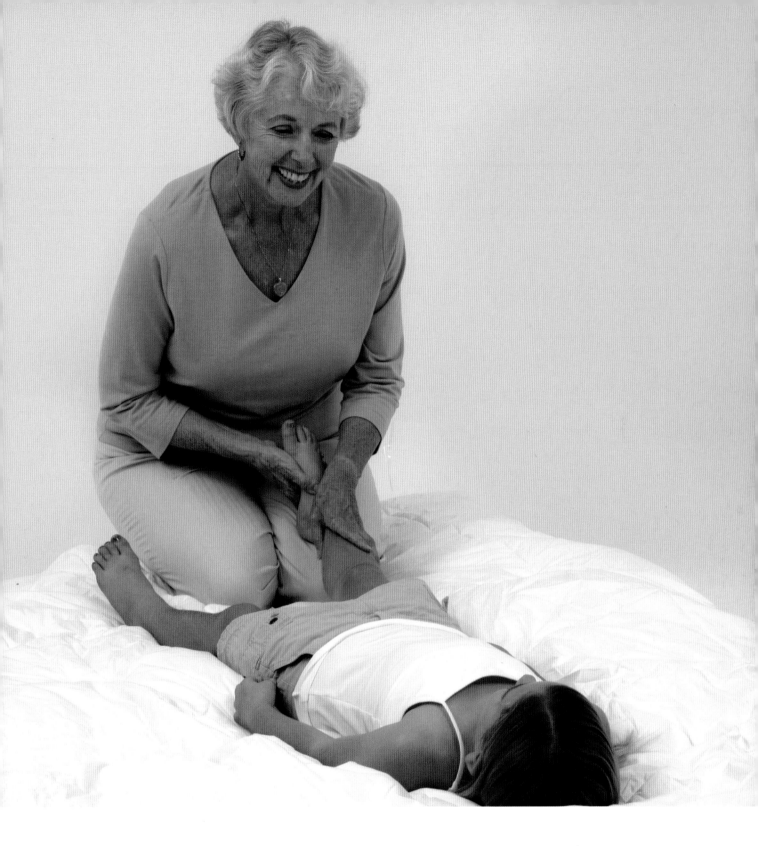

Massage is the gift that keeps on giving. Apply the three principles of Touch Communications Home Massage and you will never go wrong.

# THE ARMS AND HANDS

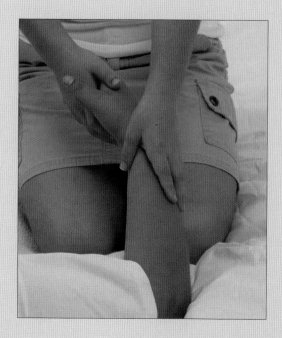

Many of us do work that requires the excessive use of our arms and hands. The list of jobs where people are constantly using their arms and hands is long—dentist, beautician, cashier, and anyone using the computer for long periods of time.

The arm and hand massage is very easy to do, and it can be done as part of a full body massage or separately within five to ten minutes. Either way, a good arm and hand massage will relax a person and relieve pain. Massaging the arms and hands increases blood circulation, which can help people with arthritis. The nicest thing about a hand and arm massage is that it can be done on anyone at just about any time. People of all ages welcome the benefits of a good arm and hand massage.

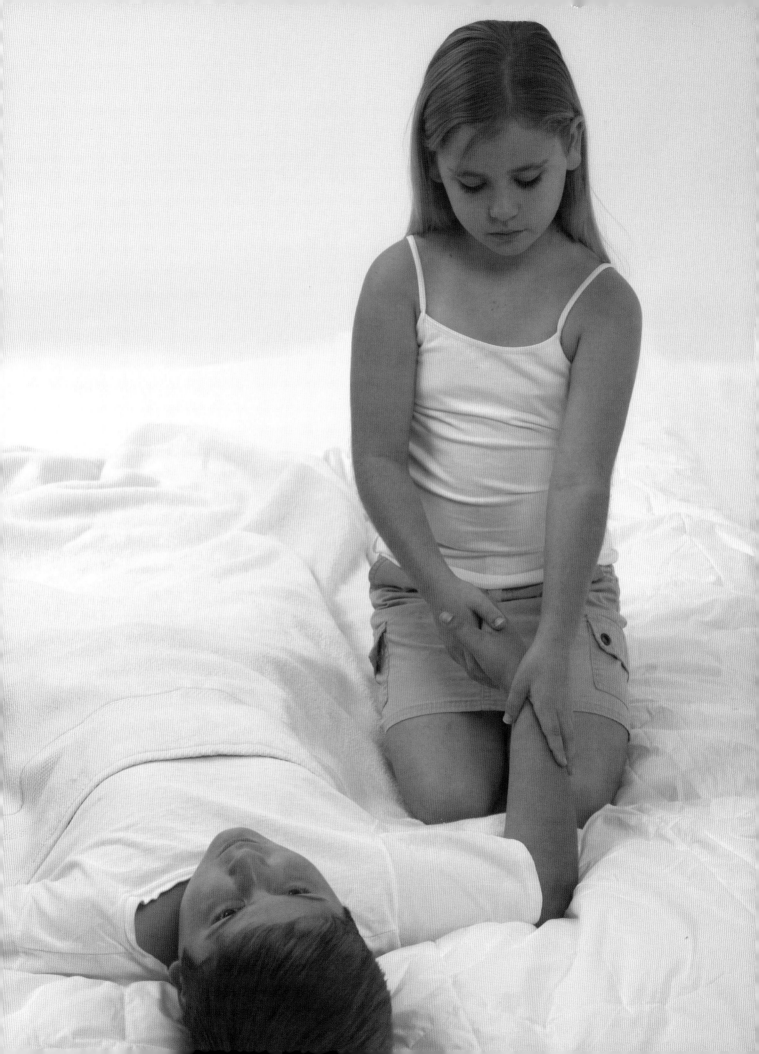

# EFFLEURAGE STROKE
## Wrist to Shoulders

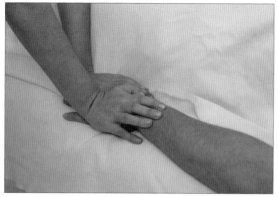 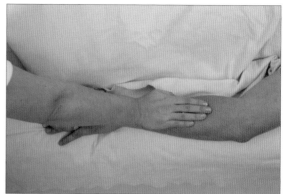

**1** Begin in the archer stance. Standing on your partner's left side, gently hold your partner's left hand with your left hand.

**2** Using your right hand, effleurage from the wrist up to and around the shoulder.

**3** Glide back down to the wrist and repeat. Use long fluid strokes. Maintain whole hand contact, with your hand conforming to your partner's arm. This stroke is often used to initiate and complete the massage routine on the arm. Repeat this stroke several times.

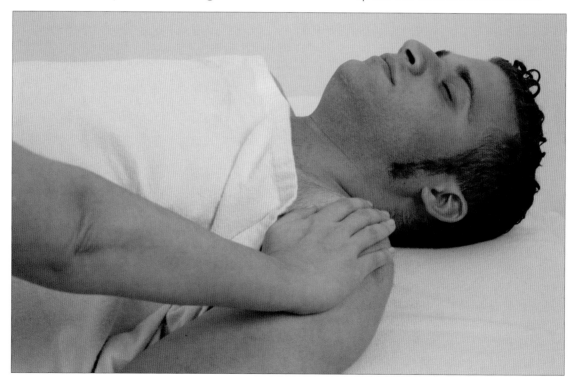

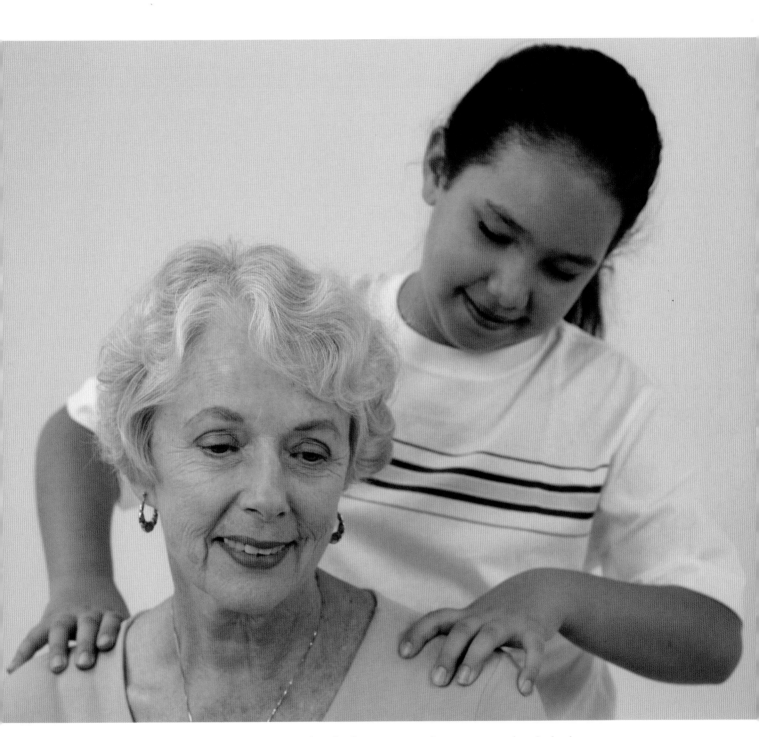

Enjoy massage as both the giver and receiver with a light heart
and the spirit of a child. Let massage be fun. Practice the strokes and routines,
but never make massage a stressful experience.
Massage should always be joyful, loving, and positive.

# EFFLEURAGE STROKE
## Back of Arm

There are times when you only work on the back of the body. This stroke can be used to massage the arm while your partner is lying face down.

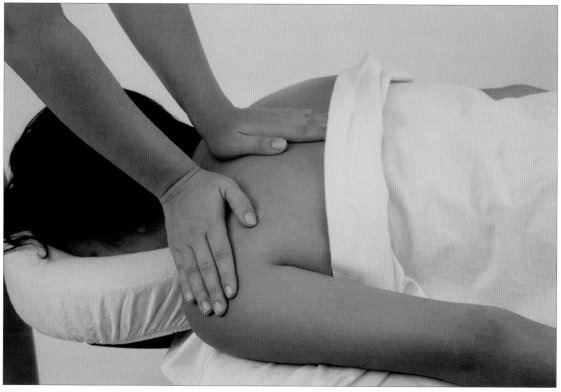

**1** Standing at your partner's head, place both palms on his shoulders. With full contact, glide one hand out towards the top of the arm. Keep gentle contact with your other hand.

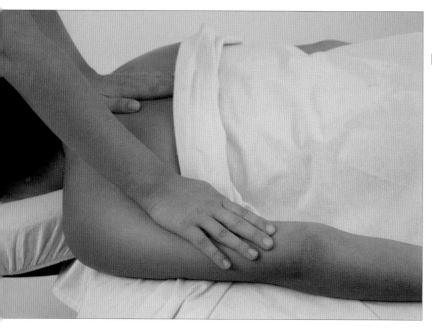

**2** Effleurage down the arm to the wrist. Glide over the elbow but do not apply pressure to the elbow.

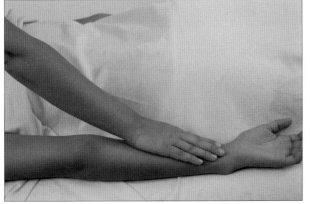

**3** Increase the pressure and continue the stroke down the forearm, over the hand and off the fingers. Lift your hand, place it back on the shoulder and repeat the effleurage stroke. On the last stroke, end on your partner's hand and hold for five seconds.

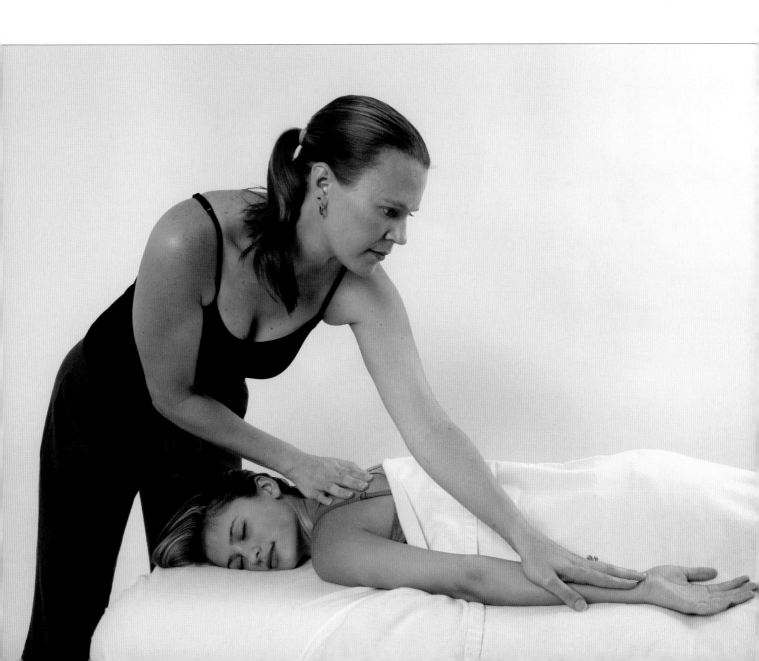

# THUMB CIRCLING STROKE
## Back of Hand

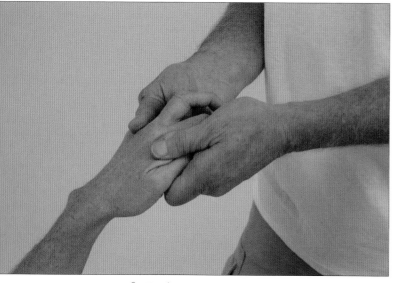

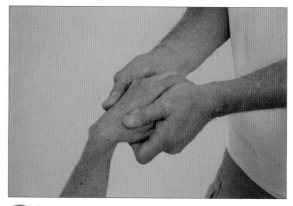

**2** Start at the base of the fingers and begin making circles over the tendons to the outside of the hand. Move slowly and apply firm pressure as you work up to the wrist.

**1** Facing the head of the table, hold your partner's hand in your hand with your fingers on the bottom of the hand and your thumbs on top.

# THUMB CIRCLING STROKE
## Palm of Hand

**2** Continue this stroke up the hand to the wrist. Remember that massage routines are not carved in stone. (If you get the notion, work your thumbs beyond the hand and up the arm).

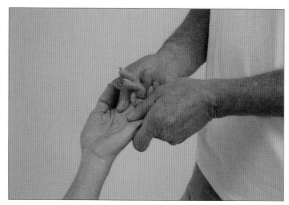

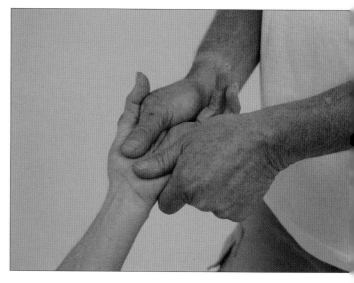

**1** For this stroke, your thumbs should be in the palm of your partner's hand. Start at the base of the fingers and glide outward from the center of the hand.

# COMPRESSION AND STRETCHING STROKE
## Fingers and Thumbs (Digits)

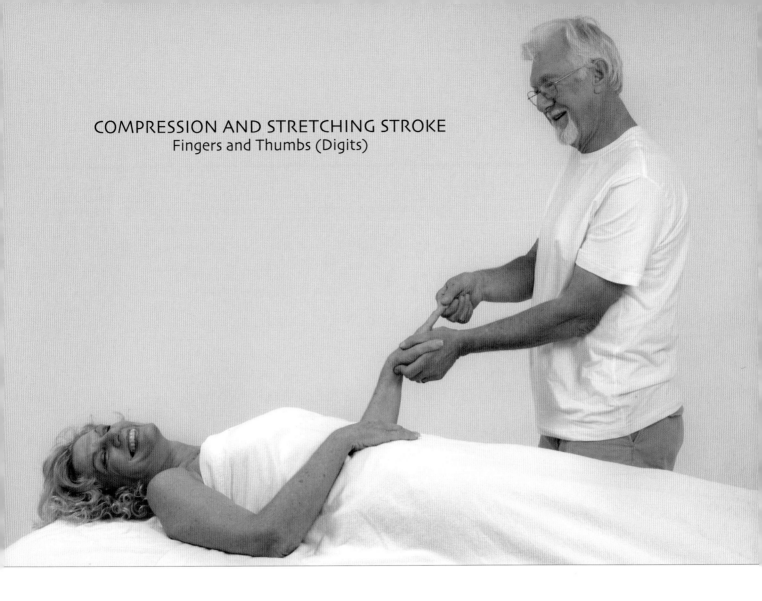

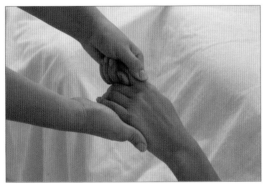

1 Gently hold your partner's hand. With your thumb and index finger, begin near the knuckle and do gentle squeezes out to the fingertip. When you reach the tip of the finger, pull (extend) the digit, hold for five seconds and slowly release.

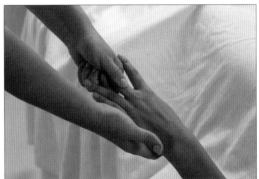

2 Begin with the little finger and with an even flow do one digit, then move on to the next. Be sure not to jerk the fingers.

# THE FEET

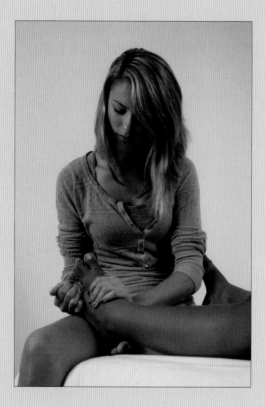

The human foot is a biological wonder. It is strong, flexible, weight-bearing and versatile. The foot is resilient and the most utilized part of our body. The average person uses their feet to move more than 100,000 miles in a lifetime. Still, we often take our feet for granted, concerning ourselves more with our appearance than the health and care of our feet.

If you have been rushing around all day, a foot massage will help restore your aching feet. The foot contains an intricate network of nerves and massaging the feet can stimulate and rejuvenate the whole body. A foot massage is also one of the most relaxing treats that you can give your partner. A foot massage can be part of a full body massage or done separately.

It is a good idea to have your partner wash and dry her feet before starting the foot massage.

# EFFLEURAGE STROKE
## Top and Bottom of Foot

This stroke can be done in either direction, from toe to ankle or ankle to toes. (For most strokes, your and your partner's comfort is more important than the direction of the stroke).

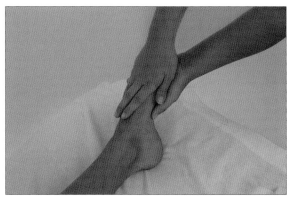

1 You can begin a foot massage by warming up the feet. Start with one hand on the top of the foot and the other hand on the bottom. Begin at the base of the toes.

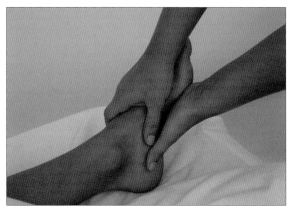

2 Move one hand followed by the other or move both hands at the same time. Continue to work up the foot to the ankle.

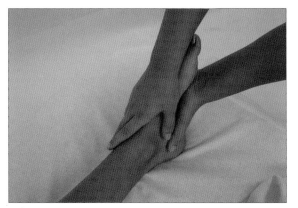

3 Use moderate pressure while molding your hand to the contour of the feet. You can repeat this stroke several times.

# THUMB CIRCLING
## Bottom of Foot

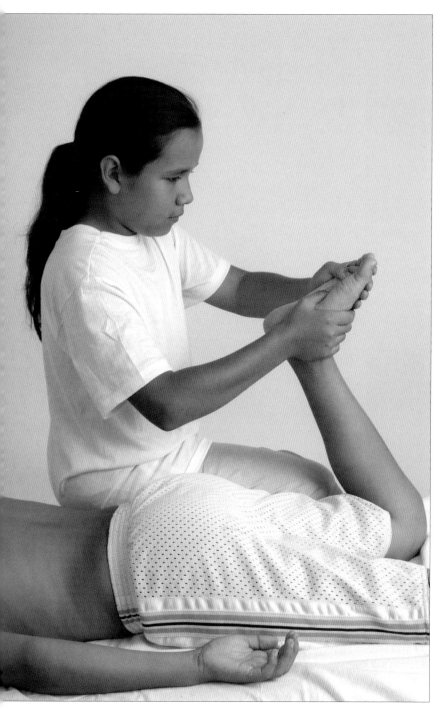

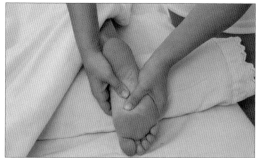

**1** Hold your partner's foot in your hands with your fingers on the top of the foot and your thumbs on the bottom. Make circles starting at the heel of the foot working all the way to the toes.

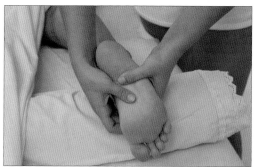

**2** You can apply firm pressure as long as you work slowly and deliberately.

# THUMB EFFLEURAGE STROKE
## Top of Foot

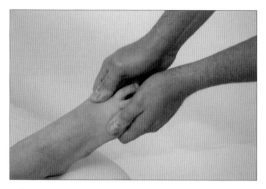

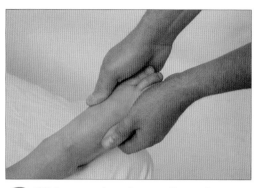

1 Start at the base of the toes with your fingers on the bottom of the foot and your thumbs on the top.

2 Glide your thumbs out from the center of the foot to each side, working your way up the foot.

# EFFLEURAGE STROKE
## Bottom of Foot

# COMPRESSION AND STRETCHING STROKE
## Toes

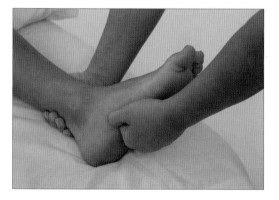

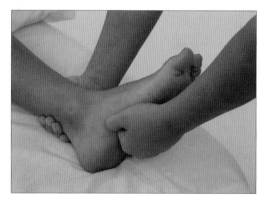

Support the foot with one hand. Place the other hand on the bottom of the foot and curl your fingers so you are gliding down the foot with your knuckles. This is a firm stroke. Keep your hands soft and conform them to the contour of the foot. (You can lean your body in to the foot to increase pressure, instead of taking it in your back.)

Gently support your partner's foot. With your thumb and index finger, clasp the base of the toe and do gentle squeezes out to the tip of the toe. When you reach the end of the toe, pull (stretch) the toe, hold for five seconds, and then slowly release. Massage all toes, one by one.

# THE ABDOMEN

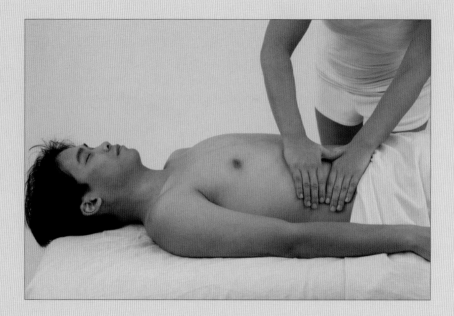

Before you begin the massage, ask your partner if he or she wants work on the abdomen. Some people feel vulnerable and apprehensive about being massaged on the abdomen. But those willing to accept the work will find it especially enjoyable, comforting, and relaxing.

Abdominal massage can improve the circulation of blood and lymph and stimulate the movement of the small intestines. It can relieve constipation. Massaging the abdomen soothes away stomach aches, indigestion and can help relieve bad menstrual pains.

It is especially important for the giver of the massage to be very centered, relaxed, and comfortable when massaging the abdomen. All of your movements should be gentle, slow, and done with great care.

# HAND ON HAND CIRCLING STROKE
## Abdomen

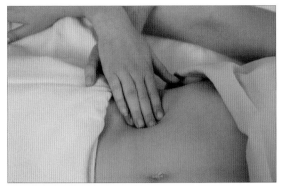

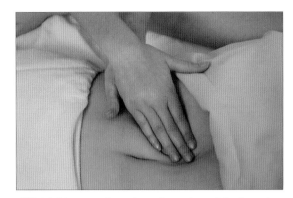

1 Position yourself on the right side of your partner. Place one hand on the other and gently lay them on the right side of the belly with your palms facing down.

2 With your hands soft and molded to the tissue, begin making a circle going clockwise.

3 Continue the circle to the left side of the abdomen. Keep sweeping your hands over the abdomen in a circular motion until you have completed a full circle.

4 Repeat this stroke several times. Apply moderate pressure. Stay present and relaxed in your own body as you work the abdomen.

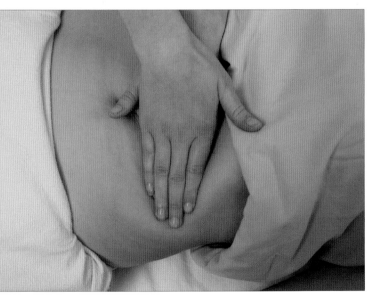

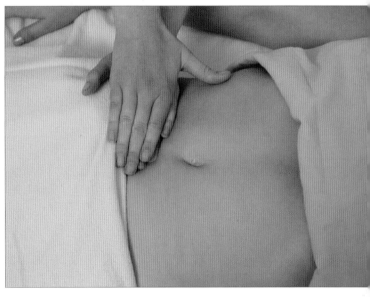

## EFFLEURAGE STROKE
### Abdomen and Waist

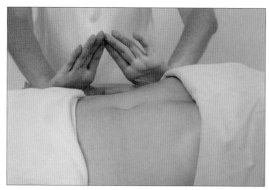

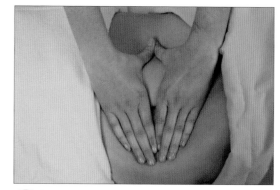

**1** Position yourself on the right side of your partner. In preparation for this stroke, open your hands, cross your thumbs, and bring your index fingers together.

**2** Bring your thumbs softly against your partners right waist. Use soft, firm pressure as you glide your hands over the abdomen. Make sure that your hands are soft and that they are conforming to the shape of the body.

**3** Reach under the waist on the opposite side. With your hands soft, clasp the tissue and slowly move back to where you began this stroke. You can repeat this stroke several times. Always massage the belly with a great deal of respect and presence.

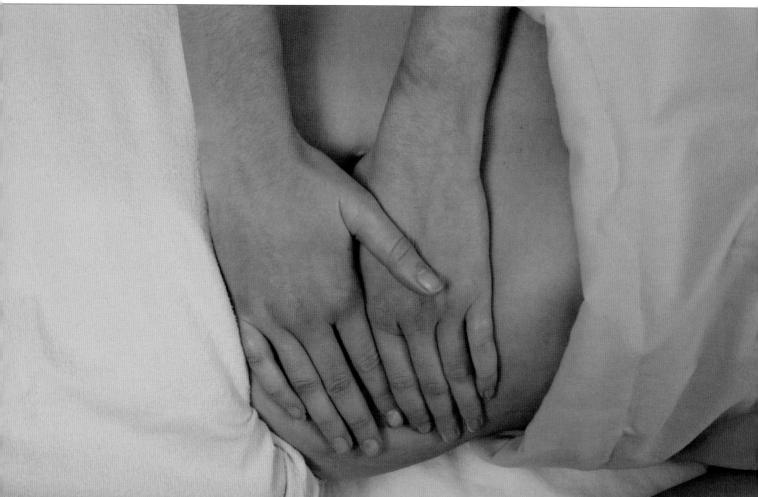

# EFFLEURAGE AND STRETCHING STROKE
## Waist

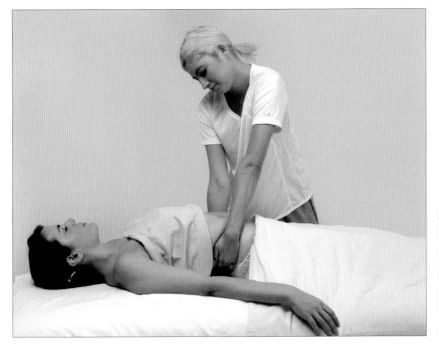

**1** Position yourself so you are comfortable. Gently slide both hands under your partner's waist as far as you can reach with your palms facing up and your fingers pointing towards each other.

**2** Slowly pull, lift, and stretch the waist by moving your hands from the back of the waist towards the navel. Do not make any sudden movements. You can repeat this stroke several times. This stroke opens the area between the pelvis and ribs.

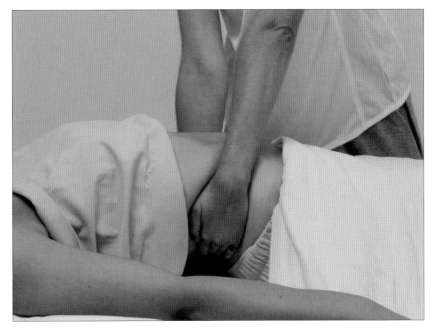

# THE HEAD AND NECK

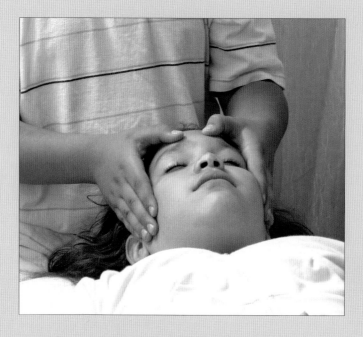

A good head, neck, and shoulder massage is a delight anytime. When giving a full-body massage, adding a head massage is the icing on the cake and can bring a deep sense of calm and well-being to the receiver.

Working at a desk or computer all day long can lead to a great deal of tension being stored in the upper body, especially our neck and shoulders. Many of us have poor posture or work in professions that have us slouching our shoulders for long periods of time, creating a lot of tension in our entire body. Massage can release those tight areas and remind us what relaxation feels like.

Make the last four or five minutes of a head, neck, and shoulder massage slow, smooth, and rhythmic.

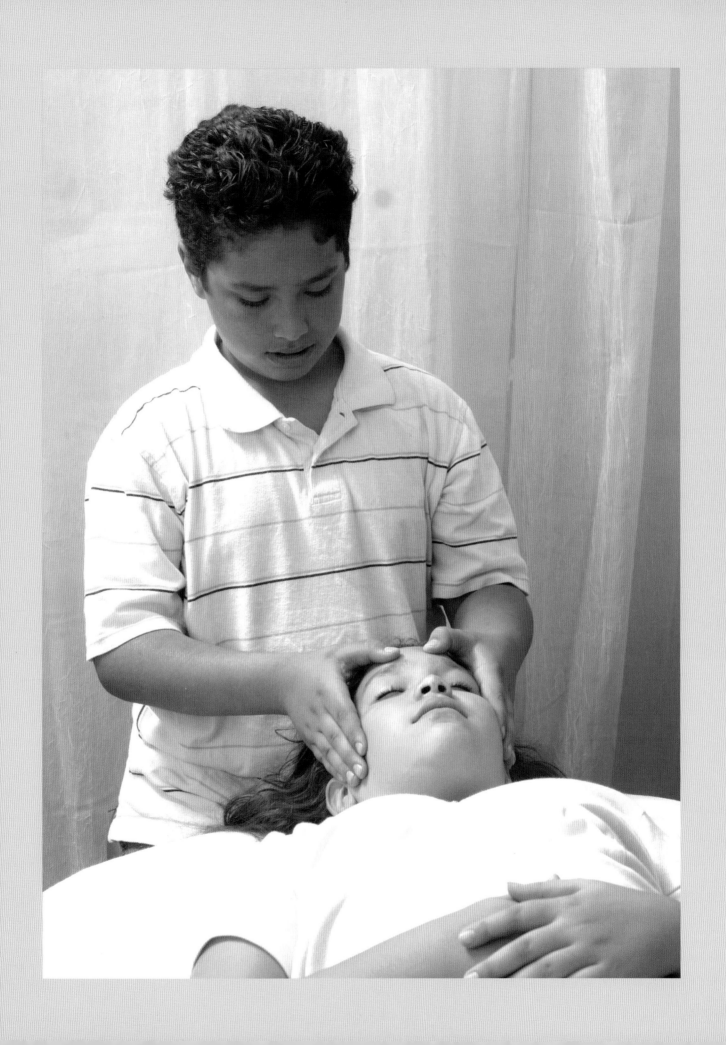

# EFFLEURAGE STROKE
## Head, Neck, and Shoulders

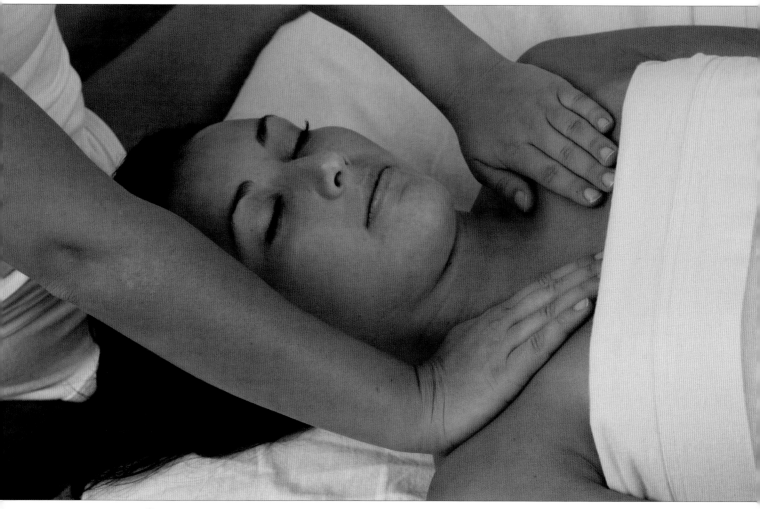

1 This effleurage stroke is done in one full, sweeping motion. Start with your hands next to each other just below the collar bones (the wing-shaped bones just below the neck) at the base of the neck.

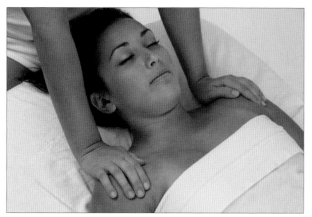

2 Keeping your hands soft and molded to the contour of the shoulders, apply smooth but firm pressure as you fan your hands out and behind around the shoulders. Your hands should end palms up.

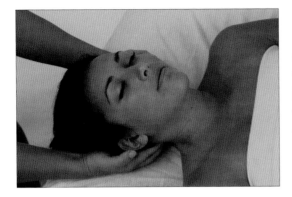

**3** Glide the pads of your fingers along the muscles of the shoulders and up the back of the neck to the occipital ridge (the groove at the back of the head where the base of the skull meets the spine). Gently remove your hands from under the head and begin again.

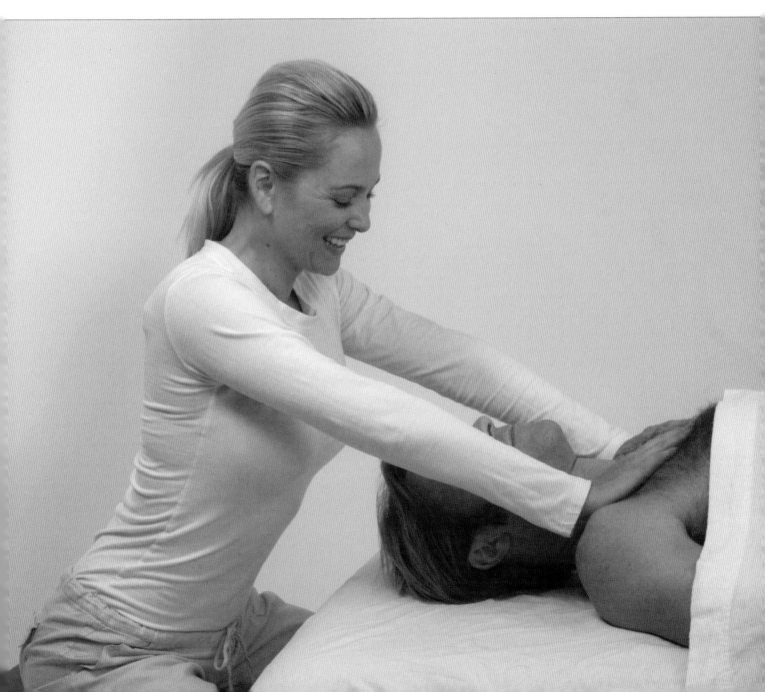

# COMPRESSION AND STRETCHING STROKE
## Neck and Shoulders

1 Place your hands gently on the head be-hind the ears. Rotate the head to the left without lifting it. Place your left hand in back of the head with your fingers between the groove of the head and the neck. Place your right hand on your partner's right shoulder and gently stretch the neck by pushing the shoulder down towards the toes with your right hand. Hold for five seconds and slowly release. Repeat this stroke several times.

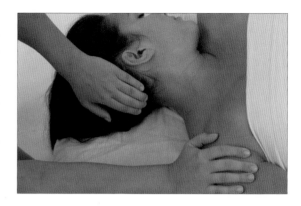

2 Turn your partner's head to center and then to the right side. Place your right hand in the back of the head with your fingers between the groove of the head and the neck and your left hand on your partner's left shoulder. With your left hand gently stretch the neck by compressing the shoulder down towards the toes. Hold for about five seconds and release slowly. Repeat this stroke several times.

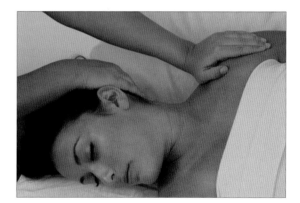

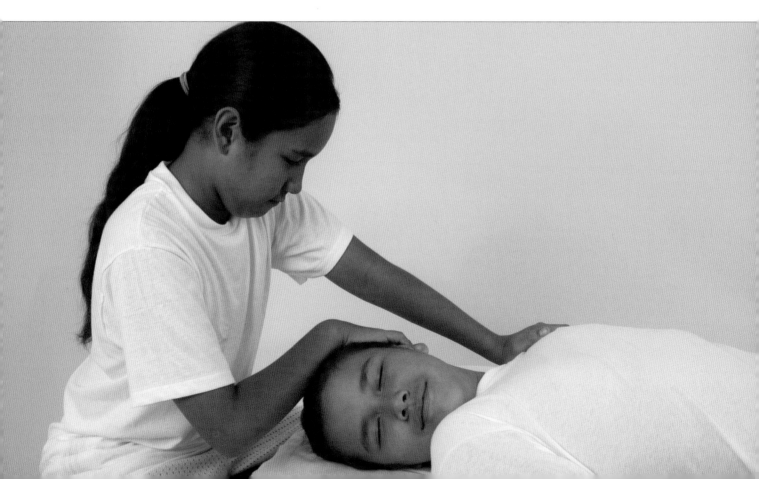

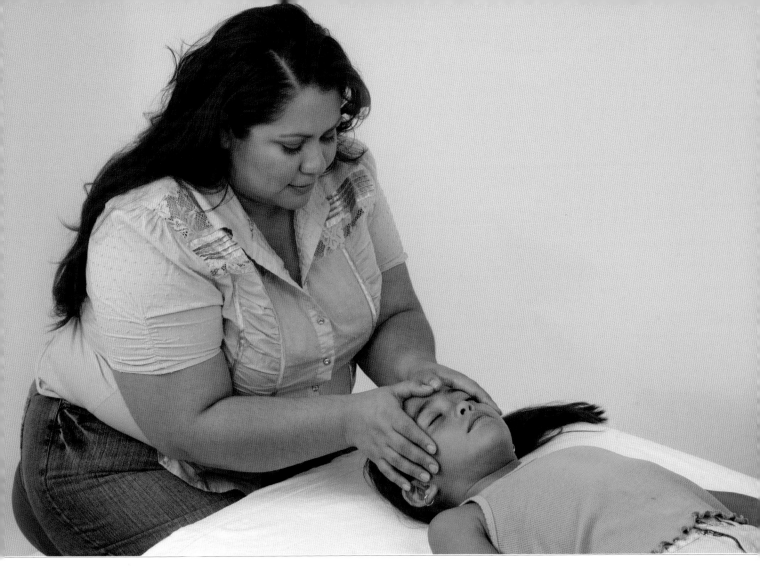

## EFFLEURAGE STROKE
### Forehead

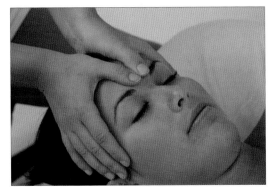

**1** Place your thumbs gently on the center of the head with the tips of your thumbs on the eyebrow bone. Your fingers should be resting gently on the sides of your partner's head.

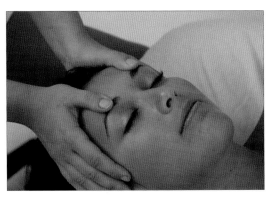

**2** Next, glide your thumbs apart and to the sides. Keep full, firm contact with your thumbs.

# STRETCHING STROKE
## Head and Neck

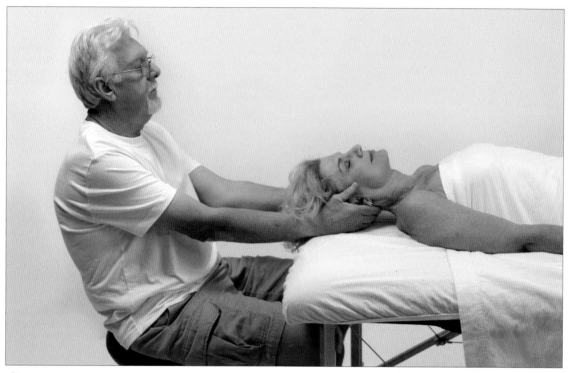

Clasp your hands around the base of the skull with your fingers in the groove between the head and the neck. Slowly lean back with your body weight, hold for four or five seconds and release slowly. You can repeat this stroke several times.

# CIRCLING STROKE
## Scalp

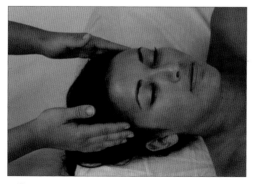

**1** Using the pads of your fingers and thumbs, make slow and deliberate circling moves on the scalp. You can start by making circles at the front and work over the whole head. Do extra work at the hollows at the base of the skull.

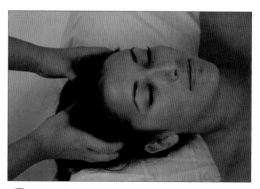

**2** Continue working the scalp. You can use the pads of your thumbs as well as the pads of your fingers. Rather than sliding your fingers over the scalp, move the scalp around to release tension in the underlying muscles. Relax your own body while you work.

# GENTLE TOUCH STROKE
## Head and Heart

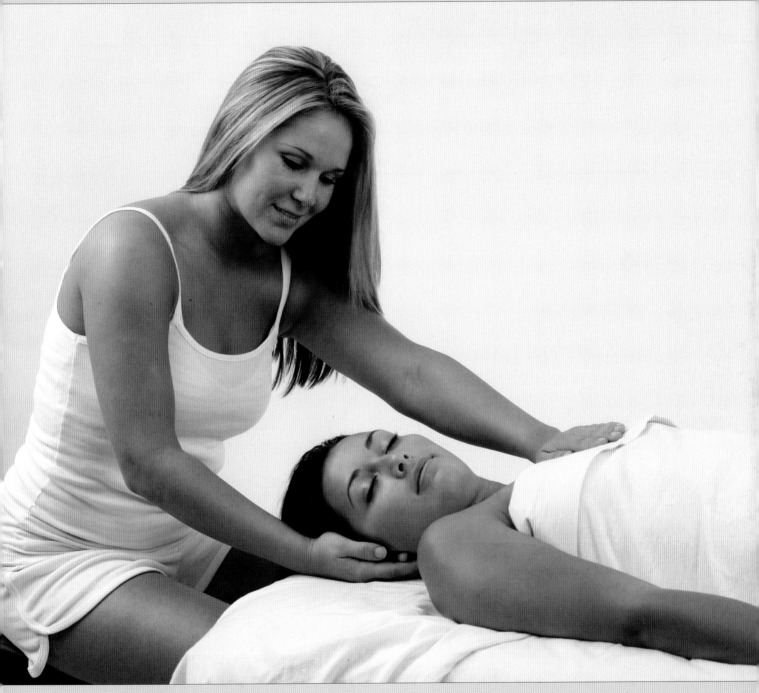

This is an excellent stroke to use to end a massage. Place one hand on the heart and one behind the head, or place your hands gently on your partner's shoulders. Remain there for 20 to 30 seconds. Breathe slowly and relax your hands and body. Let your partner rest and absorb all the sensations. Then gently remove your hands. This will signal the close of the massage.

# SECTION THREE

# BRINGING HOME MASSAGE
# INTO YOUR LIFE

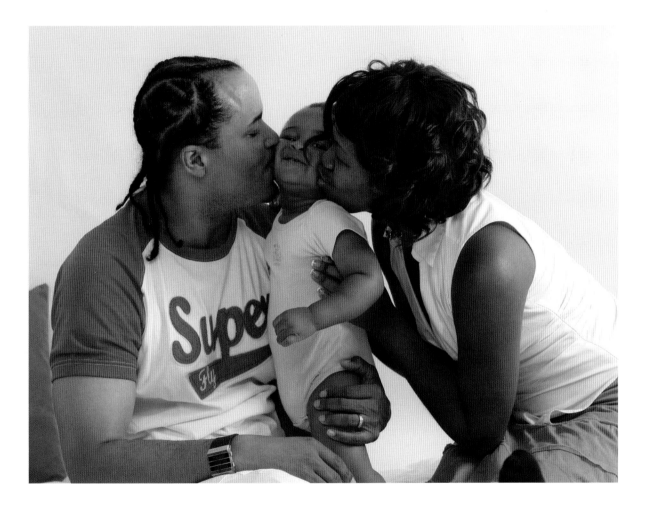

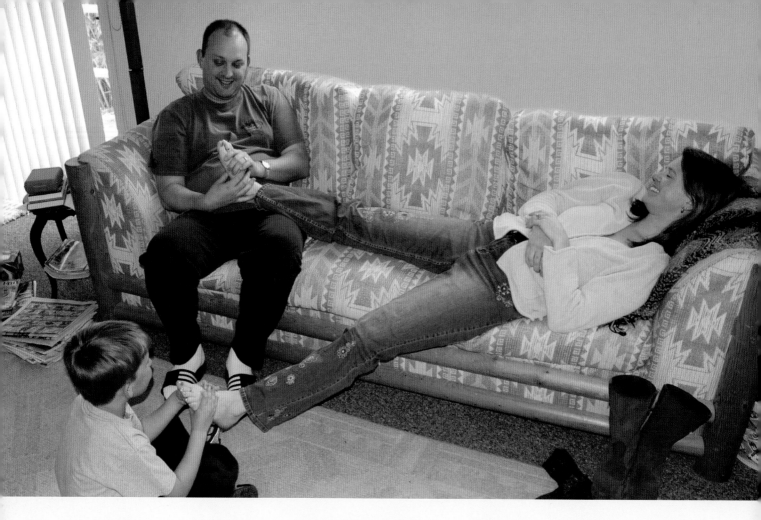

## CHAPTER EIGHT

# FAMILY

To put the world right in order, we must first put the nation in order;
to put the nation in order, we must first put the family in order;
to put the family in order, we must first cultivate our personal life;
we must first set our hearts right.

—Confucius

# A NATURAL EXPRESSION

Massage is transforming family life. Families report fewer fights, more laughter, better health, and increased relaxation. They find that they spend less time watching television and on the computer and more time on the massage table, connecting with one another.

Home massage should be a fun, loving, and joyful time. Create an atmosphere in the home that is comfortable with touch. Sharing massage in the home allows parents to model proper touch with their children. Make massage a natural expression for every family member.

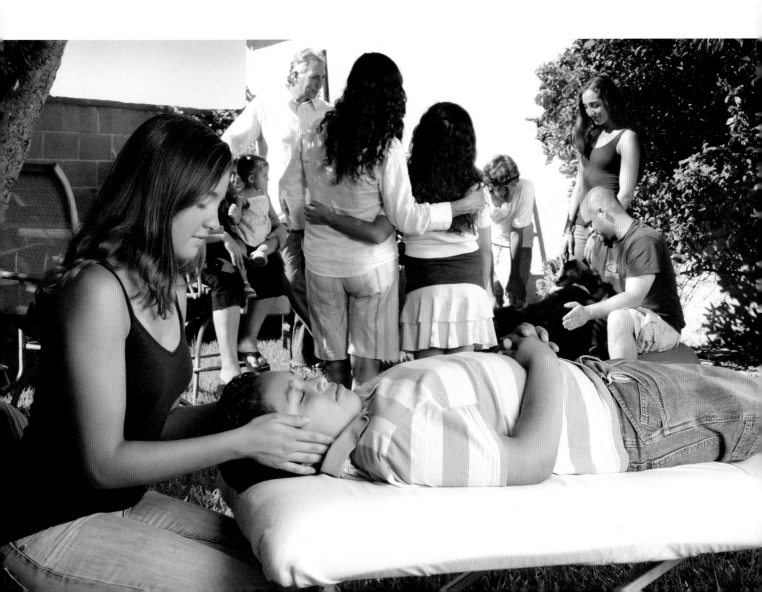

# MASSAGE IDEAS FOR THE FAMILY

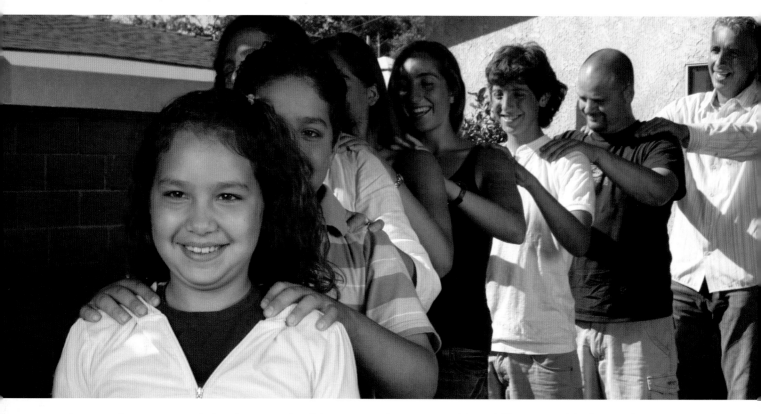

A massage train is an easy and quick way to rejuvenate and bond. Sit or stand in front of each other and rub the other's back. Have the caboose become the engine every few minutes.

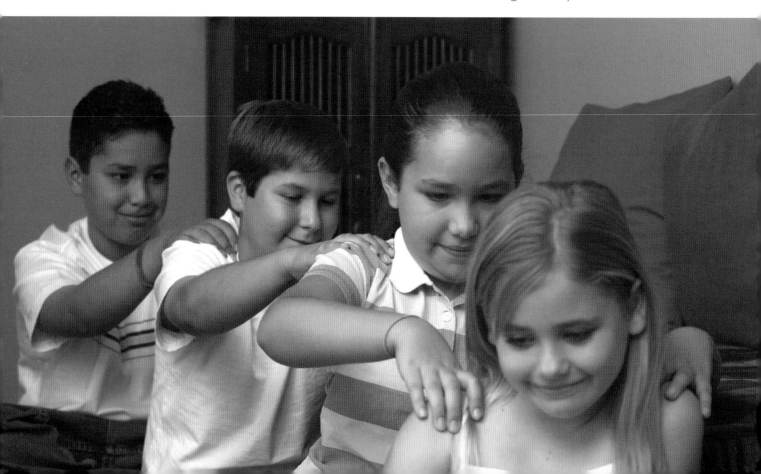

Encourage everyone in the family to make up their own massage moves. Think of the receiver's body as a "blank canvas" and paint a picture that says relaxation and health.

Set aside a Family Night. Turn off all cell phones, televisions, and computers. Take turns giving and receiving. The massage can be 10 minutes each or longer.

Make a weekly appointment to share massage with any family member. This weaves massage into the fabric of family life. Children and parents look forward to this special time to relax and connect with one another.

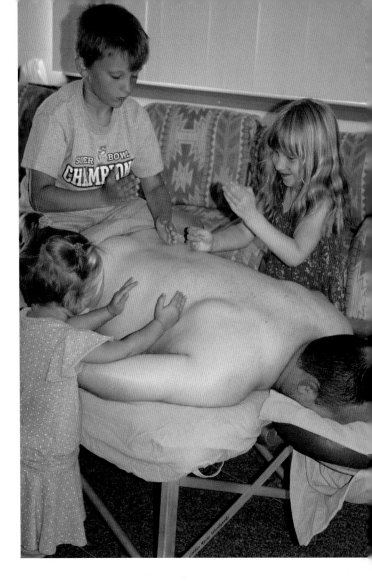

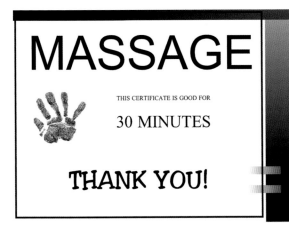

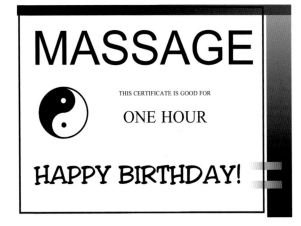

Offer each other a gift certificate for massage.
It can be given as a reward, birthday present, or in exchange for chores.

# PREGNANCY

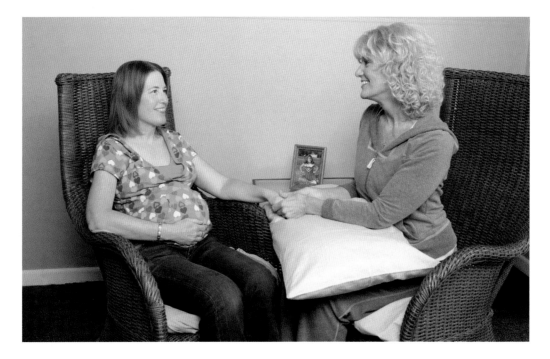

Massage is a wonderful gift to give a pregnant spouse or family member. Massage soothes nerves and alleviates common complaints of pregnancy such as backaches, shoulder tension, and aching legs and feet. It is also a wonderful way for the mother and father to stay involved during the pregnancy. Gentle, calming strokes stimulate the circulation without putting strain on the heart and can help reduce blood pressure, calming both the mother and child.

## MASSAGE DURING PREGNANCY

Reduces stress and insomnia

Eases tension on weight-bearing muscles

Reduces swelling from an increase in blood and lymphatic circulation

Reduces muscle cramps, spasms, and myofascsial pain,
    especially in the lower back, neck, hips, and legs.

Enhances the pliability of skin and the underlying tissue

Reduces the physical and emotional strains of mothering

Reduces labor pains

Provides emotional support and nurturance

Reduce swelling in hands and feet

Relieves headaches and sinus congestion

Positioning during a massage is critical to the safety and well-being of both the mother and the baby. Set up the massage table so the receiver will lie in a semi-reclining position. This is not only comfortable, but also safe for the baby. Turn the pregnant person from side to side to do her back and hips. You can use body pillows, wedge pillows, and extra padding for added comfort. Remember to be very gentle, especially on the abdomen and lower back. Avoid using deep pressure and percussive strokes. Some massage therapists suggest refraining from massage during the first trimester, but many women find gentle strokes very calming during this sometimes physically and emotionally challenging phase of their pregnancy. Checking with the woman's doctor is always the best course of action.

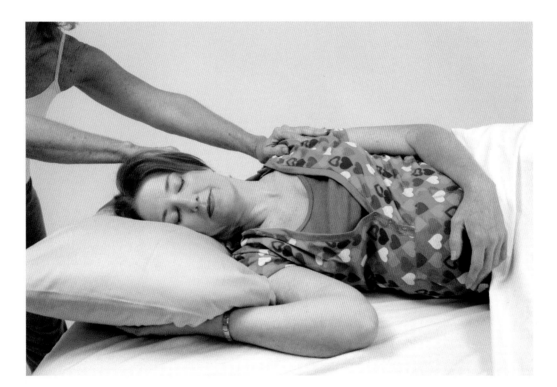

Twenty-six pregnant women were assigned either to a massage therapy group or a relaxation therapy group for five weeks. Only the massage group reported improved mood, better sleep, and less back pain by the last day of the study. Also the massage therapy group had decreased uterine stress-hormones levels, and experienced fewer complications during labor, post-natal problems with their infants, and premature births.[13]

# ILLNESS

If a drug were discovered that provided the many benefits massage gives, pharmaceutical companies would be falling all over themselves to bottle it. Granted, pharmacological interventions are necessary, but percodan cannot touch the pain in the soul, and prednisone can't heal wounded emotions.
— Gayle MacDonald, *Medicine Hands: Massage Therapy for People With Cancer*

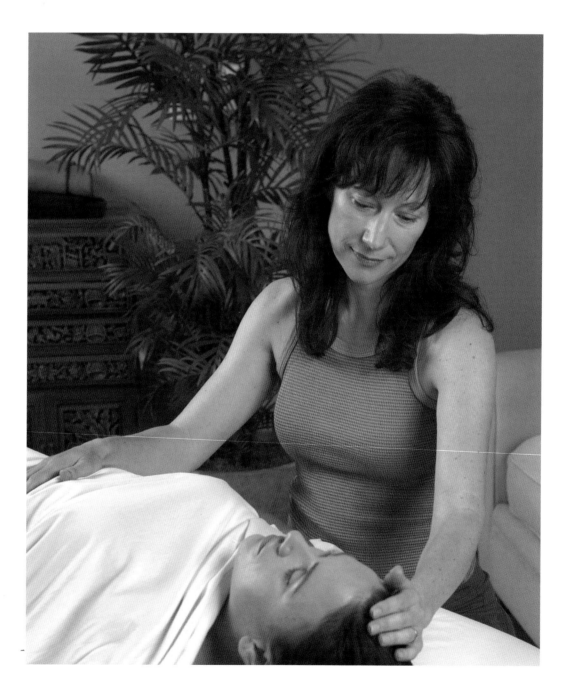

Throughout history, the healing power of touch provided relief for the ill when seeking medical care. Although medical technology has advanced, many medical professionals seem to have lost touch literally with the patient. In today's touch-phobic world, the use of hand-holding and empathetic embrace is now minimal or obsolete in doctors' offices and hospitals. Family members and friends must fill in the gap and provide this supportive, healing touch for their sick loved ones.

Sometimes we do not know what to say when someone is ill. Yet often words are not what is needed. The most basic need of a patient, sometimes more vital to them than medication, is comforting touch. When a patient's need for touch is satisfied, he or she is strengthened and better able to deal with problems and traumas.

Some of our most cherished memories of childhood are of our parents' nurturing, loving touch when we were sick. As adults, we all crave and need this same physical and emotional support when dealing with illness.

Offering a massage to a sick relative or friend can be a much-welcomed respite for them that brings comfort during illness. Massage helps people feel less isolated and alone. It releases natural pain relievers in the body that are stronger than morphine. The peace and relaxation that massage provides aids in the healing process.

Loved ones who are undergoing radiation and chemotherapy often experience fewer side effects if they receive regular massage. Gentle massage helps decrease nausea, improve sleep, lift depression, and ease fatigue. If massage is uncomfortable, then a loved one can offer the much needed human touch by holding the patient's hand or giving a loving embrace.

When massaging the sick and the grieving, we must learn we must learn the degree and duration of pressure most comfortable for them. Ask for feedback and keep the touch soft and nurturing.

Among patients with advanced cancer, 30 minutes of massage therapy resulted in immediate benefits to both pain and mood.[14] For more information on massaging those with cancer, please see the Further Reading section at the end of the book.

A head-and-neck massage resulted in improved heart-rate variability, decreases in tension-anxiety and anger-hostility, and a reduction in head pain among research participants with chronic tension-type headaches.[15]

# GRIEVING

When a loved one is grieving, touch is a powerful way to show concern and provide comfort when words are inadequate. You do not have to do a full body massage to show you care. Simply stroke the grieving relative's hand and arm or massage their face, neck, and shoulders to help release their physical and emotional tension. Even a hand gently laid on a shoulder or a loving touch to an arm can make a huge difference to someone experiencing loss.

Grief can be a single event of loss or the accumulated and unexpressed feelings of a lifetime. Little losses that we thought weren't major can build and trigger overwhelming emotions. Grief kept within can create physical illness and emotional distress. Poor sleep, headaches, backaches, increased anxiety, depression, and stomach ailments are all symptoms of grief.

Sometimes people who are grieving keep their emotions inside because they feel they are too overwhelming or powerful to express. When reaching out to loved ones who are grieving, even a gentle embrace or held hand can cause them to cry. Allow them the loving space to feel and release their emotions. A longer massage on the table can also be a gift of relaxation and comfort to a grieving loved one. Again, if they begin to cry, be loving and supportive without judgment and advice. Communicate through touch and know that you are providing a place for them to open, release, and feel comforted. As always, honor and respect the person's wishes on the table.

> Massage is a "commendable source of consolation support during the grieving process," according to recent research. The researchers noted: "Soft tissue massage appears to be a worthy, early, grieving-process support option for bereaved family members whose relatives are in palliative care."[16]

# IN A WHEELCHAIR

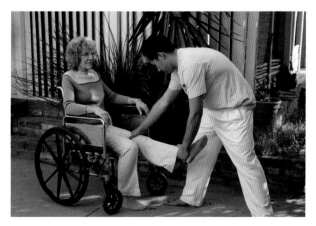

Being bound to a wheelchair, whether for a few days or a lifetime, can be physically and emotionally challenging. No matter what the reason for being in a wheelchair, seated massage can be extremely beneficial. Wheelchair massage can improve range of motion, increase circulation, and create emotional well-being.

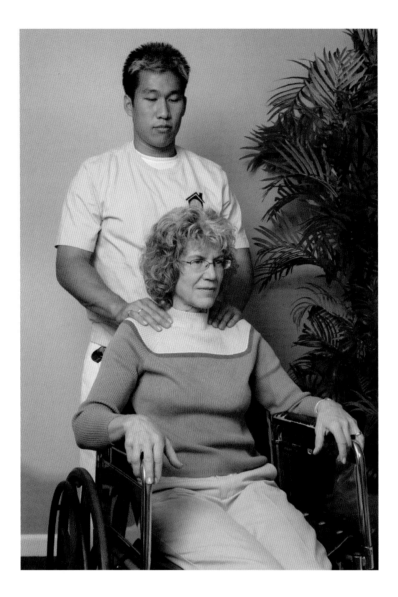

The seated position in a wheelchair can have many advantages for giving a massage. Standing behind the chair makes it easy to work on the head, neck, and shoulders, with easy accessibility to the hands and arms.

Sometimes our own discomfort or misunderstanding keeps us from reaching out with a hug or embrace to our wheelchair-bound loved ones. Being in a wheelchair can be physically and emotionally challenging. Offer your loving touch and the healing benefits of home massage.

By keeping the legs of a massage table low, those in a wheelchair can easily maneuver around the table and give a massage as well.

# PETS

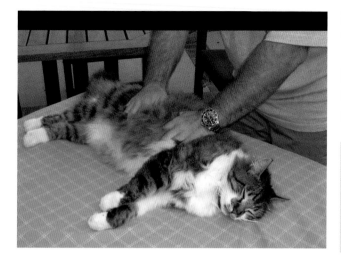

Family pets love to get on the massage table.

Pet massage is a growing modality for animal health, teaching us to support our animals and their natural need for touch.

Clinical studies have concluded that pets experience reduced pain, greater flexibility and increased circulation of both lymph and blood system with massage.[17]

# SPORTS

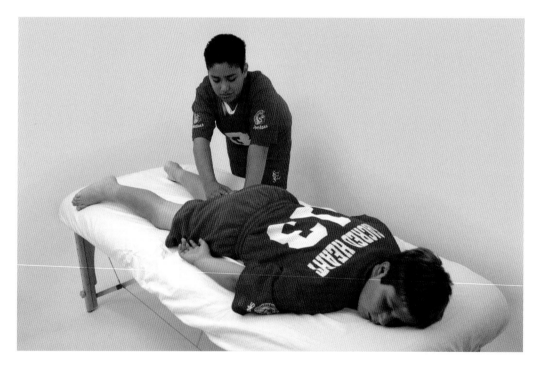

Massage is now an invaluable part of sports clinics, college athletic training, and professional locker rooms. Family members are involved in a variety of sports and exercise routines—baseball, soccer, dance, jogging, hiking, swimming, strength training, and yoga. Working out has great benefit for everyone in the family, but it can also cause stiffness, soreness and injury. Home massage is an excellent adjunct to all exercise programs, as it provides before and after care from the wear and tear of physical workouts. The convenience and availability of home massage allows us to exchange massage with family members before and after athletic events, helping to minimize injuries, increase flexibility, ease fatigue, and promote quicker recovery.

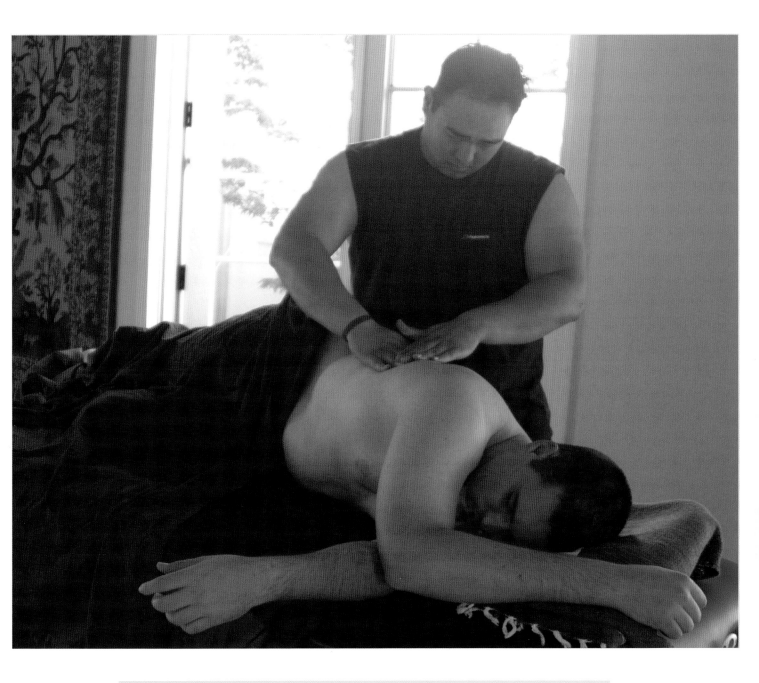

## BENEFITS OF HOME SPORTS MASSAGE

Promotes flexibility
Minimizes injuries from over-exertion
Eases fatigue
Reduces swelling
Increases blood circulation
Relieves pain

Heals strained muscles
Promotes quicker recovery
Creates peak performance
Promotes greater endurance
Reduces muscle tension

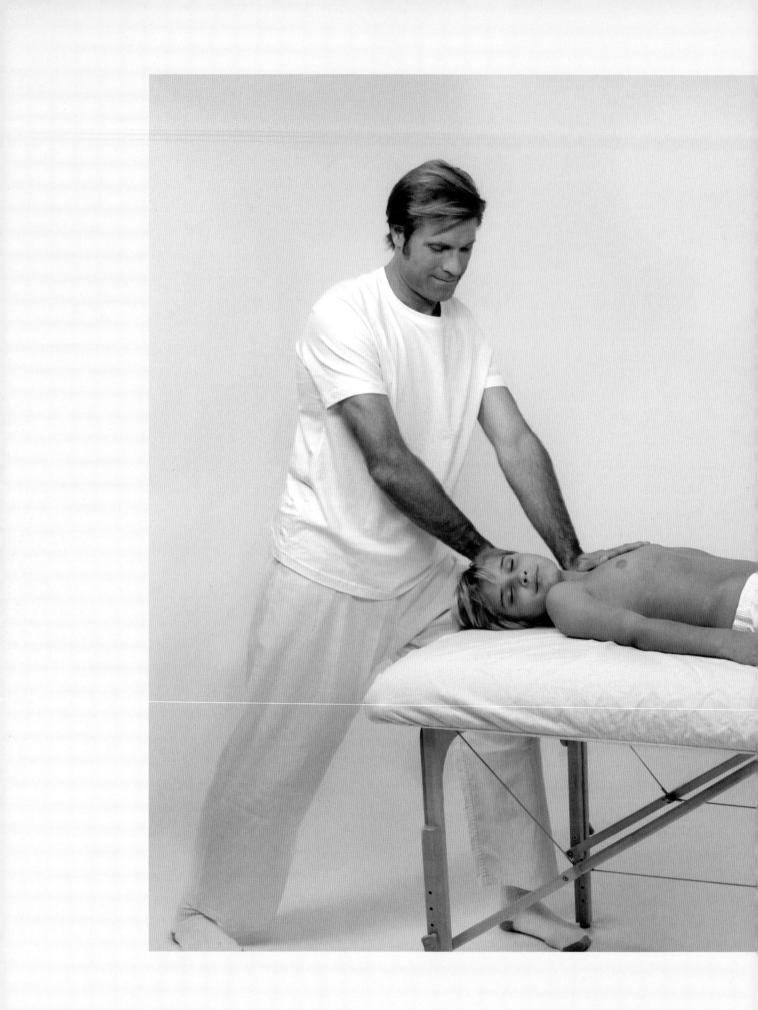

Perhaps the greatest social service
that can be rendered by anybody
to this country and to mankind is to
bring up a family.
—George Bernard Shaw

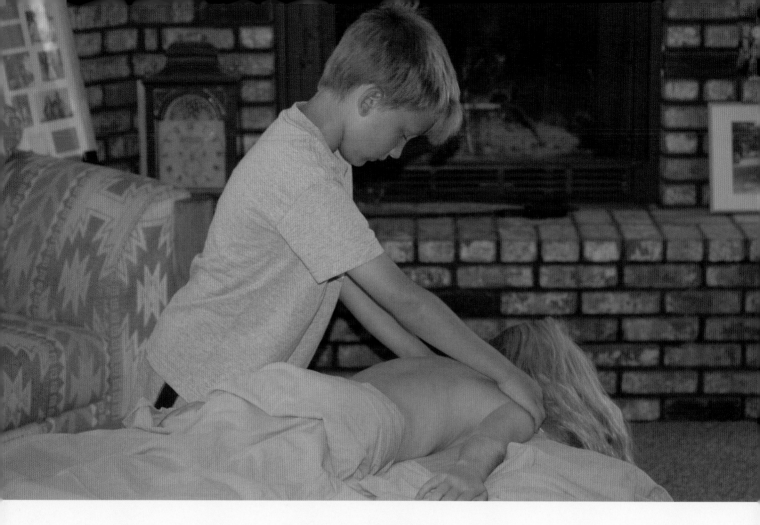

CHAPTER NINE

# CHILDREN

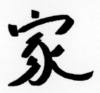

There are only two lasting bequests we can hope
to give our children. One is roots, the other is wings.

—Hooding Carter


Don't limit a child to your own understanding.
He was born in a different time.

—Rabbincal saying

As parents, we "do" for our children. We feed them, taxi them, and give them material things. But it is the hugs, pats, and embraces that children remember and cherish. Touch reassures children of their worth. Research shows that children deprived of touch grow up with a tendency towards physical violence, sleep disorders, suppressed immune systems, and impaired physical and emotional growth. Knowing through touch that they are loved gives children the strength and the foundation to deal with the stresses, strains, and insults of life.

Always remember to respect and honor your child by listening to them. Never force your touch on them.

# STRESS

Stress knows no age limits and can take its toll on children at an early age. A young toddler may feel abandoned by an absent parent. A child starting school is faced with new surroundings and classmates. Academic and social pressures are a daily part of a child's life. As children grow, healthy, spontaneous play turns into stressful, competitive sports. Years of public school change a child's natural curiosity for life into regimented learning in predetermined blocks of time. Some children are enrolled in so many activities that they lack time to just be children and enjoy creative play. Even at a young age, they are often judged more by what they achieve than who they are. In their homes, children overhear family troubles, watch disturbing images on the evening news, and are the victims of divorce.

Massaging your child and encouraging massage between siblings will give them a daily release from pent-up stress and tension. They will sleep better, increase their performance in school, and feel calm because of your loving touch.

A five-minute shoulder rub or a half-hour on the table will be a gift of physical and emotional health to your growing child.

Consistent studies of the benefits of massage therapy for children leave no doubt that massage therapy is extremely beneficial for children suffering from stress and anxiety.

Recent research found that massage therapy reduced the number, duration and severity of tension-type headaches among children ages 5 to 15 years.[18]

# GETTING A MASSAGE

Some parents, when asked how come they don't touch and hold their child, justify their lack of touch by saying, "Oh, my kid hates being touched. He runs in the opposite direction." Children who do not like to be touched are not born that way. It is a conditioned response, prompted by grownups who either refrain from touching them or hold them too tight and with too much emotional need. Sometimes we try to restrain forcibly a squirming child with hugs when they want to be doing something else. Other times we allow overbearing friends and relatives, or even strangers, to hug and kiss our children.

Children love to be touched and to touch. They are natural massage therapists. Encourage them to give and get a massage from you and foster an honoring attitude about touch.

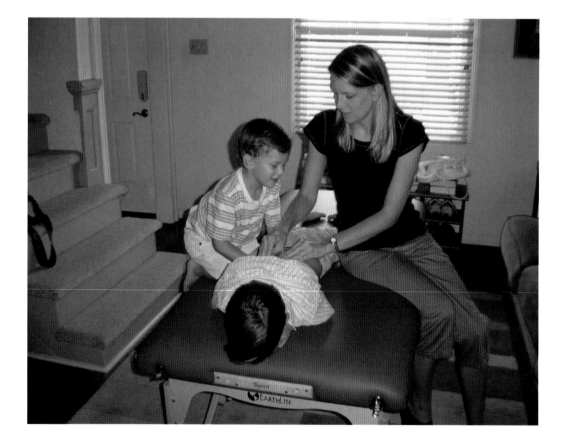

# GIVING A MASSAGE

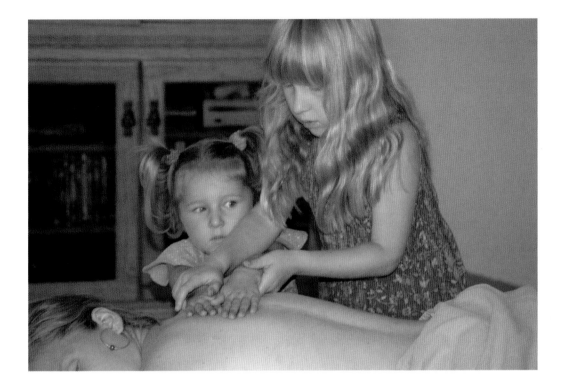

Children should be encouraged to learn massage. From the age of three onward, children are fascinated by watching massage and love to give one. They like to feel that they are doing something for someone else, making their mother or father feel good.

By five or six, many can give a really good massage. They enjoy percussion movements because they make a noise, kneading because it is like playing with clay, and stroking because it is so easy and fun.

It is easy for a young child to massage your back if they just sit or kneel on it. Just the pressure of their body on your lower back can feel wonderful.

# THE GIFT OF TOUCH TO A CHILD

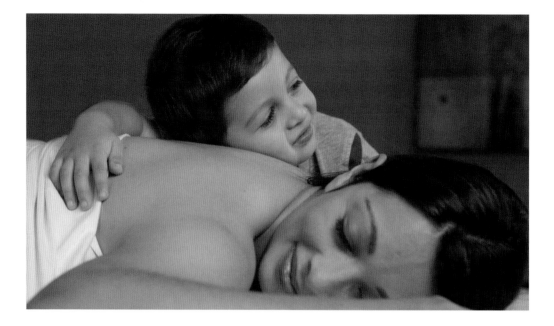

Touch is the greatest gift we can give our children. All children naturally crave touch. Children that are touched are less fearful and more secure, loving, and kind.

It is important for parents to exhibit spontaneous affection with their children. Children learn from their parents how to touch and show affection. Children learn not only from how their parents touch them but by the way their parents touch each other. They learn how to be either open and compassionate or withdrawn and defensive.

Some parents may not even realize that they are nurturing a child that will be uncomfortable with touch. Parents who were not given touch or were raised to feel uncomfortable with touch may feel like they don't know how to touch. It is important for parents to share their own touch experiences with their children, including their fears and insecurities. Exhibiting openness, vulnerability, and a desire to move past any discomfort with touch will nurture a positive relationship with touch in our children.

Loving and natural touch allows parents to connect with their children in deeper ways than words can express. The security given to children through a parent's positive, unconditional touch stays with them throughout their lifetime. They learn not only to care for themselves but also to care for others.

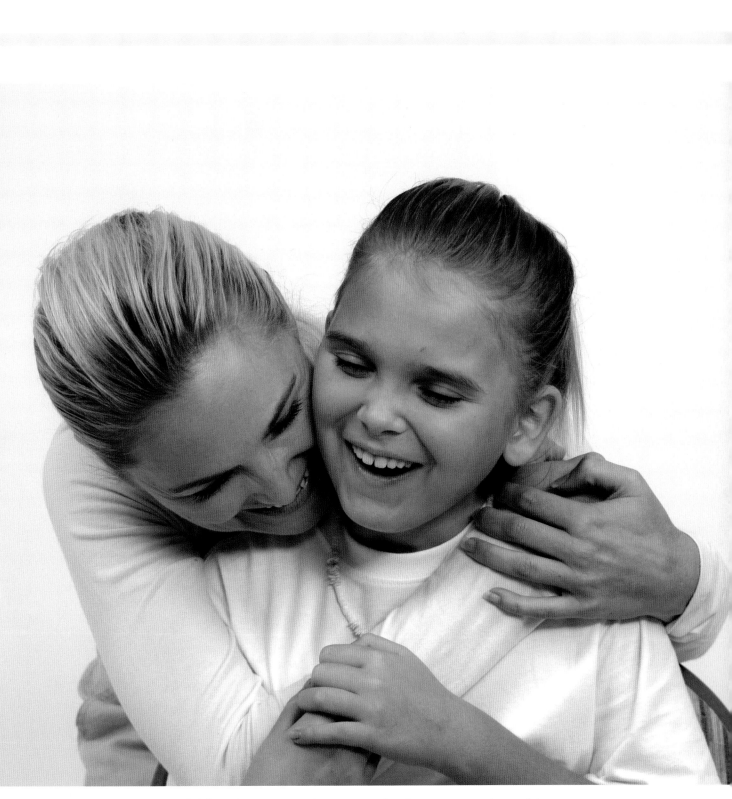

Children have never been good at listening to their elders,
but they have never failed to imitate them.

# BONDING WITH SIBLINGS

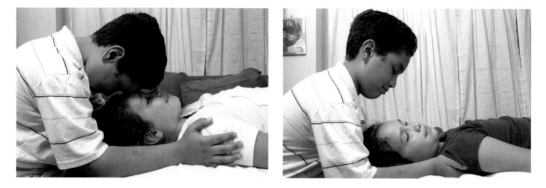

Parents of children who practice home massage have found that there is less fighting between siblings. Sharing home massage gives siblings the opportunity to nurture and be nurtured by their brothers and sisters.

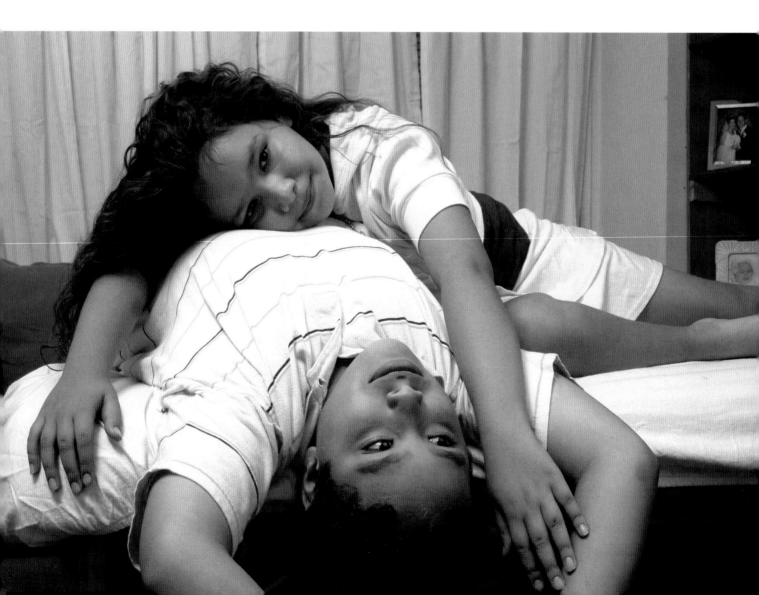

# CHILDHOOD ILLNESS

When a child is home sick with a common cold or something more serious, the healing comfort of touch will make him feel relaxed and safe. Give him a gentle massage on his face, back, arms, or legs. He will sleep better, heal faster, and be in better spirits.

Stress exacerbates the symptoms of all childhood illnesses and perhaps even causes them. Children with more serious illnesses must cope with hospitalization, painful treatments, dietary limitations, and restrictions on their normal activities. When stress hormone levels rise, symptoms increase. Massage has been found to improve blood sugar levels in childhood diabetes, improve pulmonary function in asthmatics, and improve skin conditions in children with excema.

In a study on preschool children with autism, after a 10-day period of regular massage there was a decrease in touch sensitivity, a reduction in disruptive behavior, and an increased ability to relate to their teachers.[19] In another study, parents massaged their autistic children every night. The children experienced the same benefits, along with an improvement in sleep.[20]

Parents of diabetics who massaged their children daily before bedtime reported lower anxiety and improved mood levels for both parent and child, higher insulin and food regulation scores, and decreased blood glucose levels from very high average levels to the normal range.[21]

Following one month of 20-minute bedtime massages by their parents, asthmatic children had less anxiety, an improvement in mood, and decreased stress hormones (cortisol) levels. Over the month, the children had fewer attacks and experienced improved pulmonary functioning and peak airflow.[22]

Massage therapy reduced pyschological and physical distress among children with cancer and blood diseases, thereby contributing to a general improvement in overall quality of life among subjects.[23]

# EASING A CHILD TO SLEEP

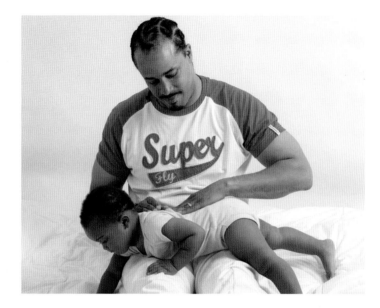

Getting children to sleep can be a draining fight in many households. Wound up from the day's activities or from a sugar overload, some children fight going to sleep. Home massage is an excellent tool to relax kids. Make a back rub part of your children's routine before going to sleep. They will be less reluctant to go to bed, sleep better, and end the day feeling your positive, unconditional love.

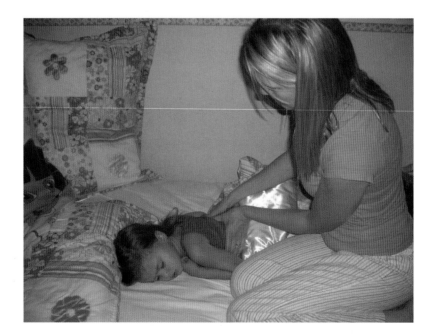

# HOMEWORK

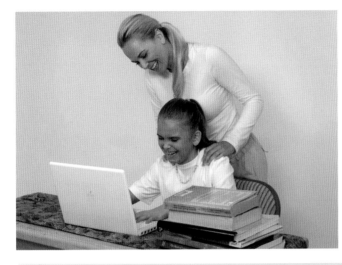

The demands of after-school homework have increased for students of all ages. They spend many hours crouched over their computers. Give your child a chair massage or a 10-minute rejuvenating break on the massage table.

Preschoolers showed better performance on tests of intellectual and manual skills after a 15-minute massage. They also slept better during naps, were calmer, and had better behavior ratings.[24]

# HYPERACTIVE CHILDREN

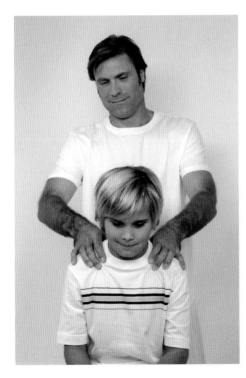

Parents of hyperactive children are all too familiar with the phrase, "Would you please just settle down?" Massage takes the same amount of time as yelling but produces incredibly better results in hyperactive children. Give your hyperactive child a mini-massage. Touch is very important to attention deficit and hyperactivity disorder children. Massage their temples, give them a shoulder rub, or lightly run your fingers through their hair to calm these children down quickly.

A study on children with attention deficit hyperactivity disorder revealed they exhibited less hyperactivity, more on-task behavior, and were happier after receiving regular massage treatments.[25]

# TEACHING CHILDREN APPROPRIATE TOUCH

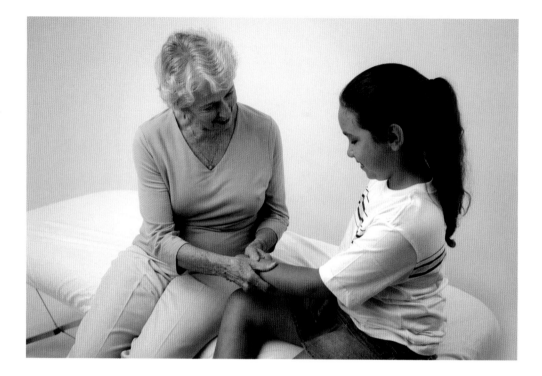

While teachers and other adults once felt comfortable patting a child on the shoulder or giving her a hug, they are now advised to avoid all physical contact for fear of misinterpretation. As parents, we must make up for this lack of touch from the world and improve our physical interactions with children at home.

How can we teach our children the dangers of improper touch without first teaching them what appropriate touch feels like? Educating children about proper touch works far better than instilling fear in children as a means to protect them from the dangers of inappropriate touch. On the table, children learn that both the receiver and the giver have the right to say no. Just as adults have the authority to say no at any time, so do children.

Home massage provides a bridge for parents to talk to their children about touch. If a parent has any doubt about any friend or family member massaging their child, they should not allow it; and if they do, they should be present during the massage. By experiencing loving, safe, and appropriate touch, children naturally learn about proper touch in the home. When kids learn to be comfortable in their bodies and can express touch in a healthy way, it positively affects all areas of their lives.

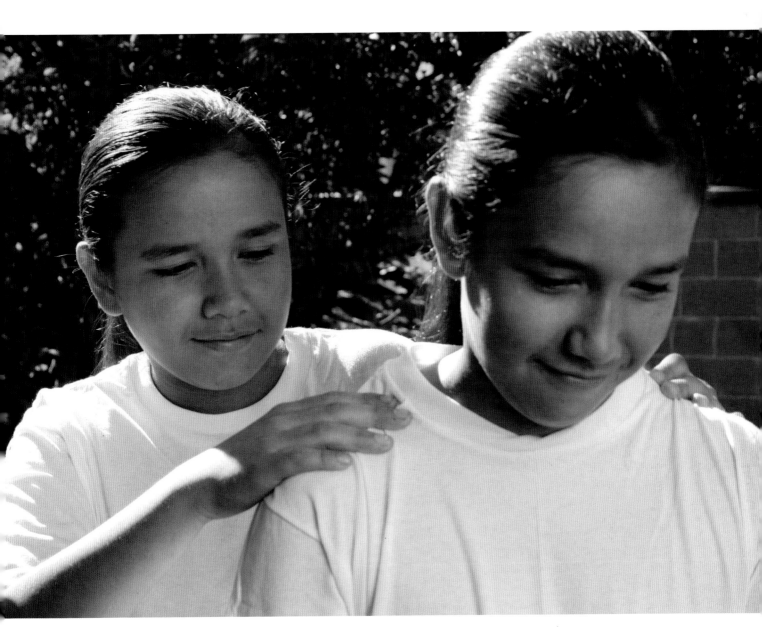

Children who learn massage are comfortable with touch
and naturally share it with their siblings.

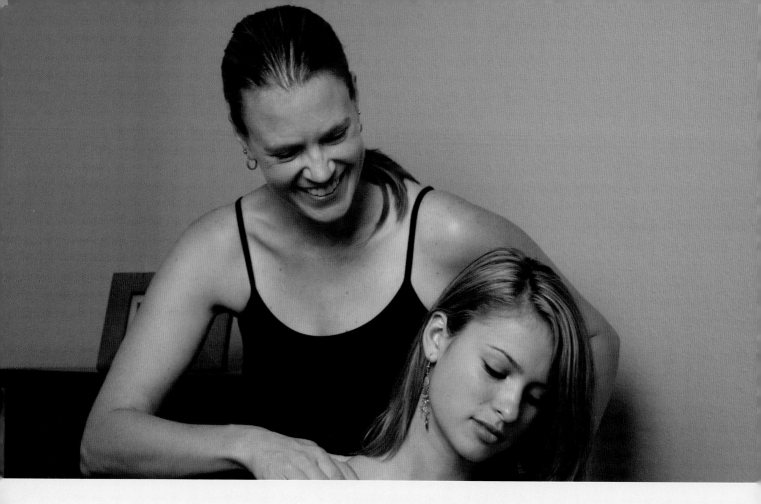

CHAPTER TEN

# ADOLESCENCE

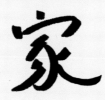

Home massage is a way to connect with your teenager
during this turbulent age.

Adolescence is one of the most difficult stages of our lives. During this dynamic period, teenagers not only encounter awkward physical changes but they also have the added expectation of approaching adulthood, which creates emotional stress and conflict. One-third of American teens have reported that they suffer from stress-related symptoms—insomnia, anxiety, and depression—daily. The remaining two-thirds experience symptoms at least once a week.

Teenagers sometimes shut down their emotions as a method of coping with the unpredictability and change in their lives. Sometimes they become irritable, angry, or resort to drugs and alcohol as a way to cope. Parents can have a difficult time adjusting to the changing moods of their teenage children.

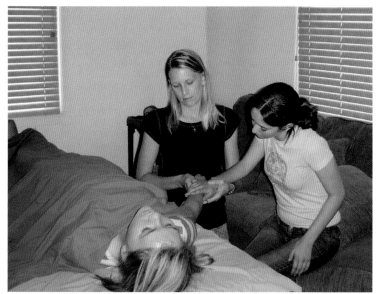

While teens may be reluctant to get or give a massage, there are plenty of reasons why this age group should be encouraged to give it a try.

Massage is good for a teenage body in the midst of rapid growth and development. Strains from competitive sports, stress from erratic sleep and overloaded schedules, and nutritional challenges from a less-than-optimal diet are all part of adolescence.

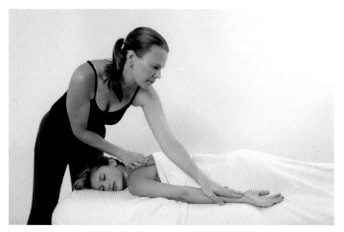

Massaging your teen can help improve body image, increase sleep, and decrease depression, stress, and anxiety.

# CONNECTING WITH YOUR TEEN

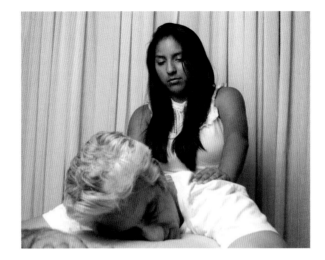

Parents with the best intentions feel trapped in their own uncertainty about how to deal with the changes going on with their adolescent children. Home massage is a way to connect with your child during this often turbulent age. If children are raised being comfortable with touch, that sense of comfort will naturally carry over into adolescence. Home massage creates a comfortable environment to discuss proper and improper touch, and other sensitive issues, with your teenager.

Adolescents crave intimacy but often look for it in the wrong places. By the time they reach junior high, they receive only half the touch they did during their younger years. The touch they do receive is now different—shoulder to shoulder and elbow to elbow—rather than hand contact. If they experience touch in the home through the natural connection of massage, they are not likely to seek dangerous and unhealthy avenues for emotional and physical contact, succumbing to peer pressure and experimenting with drugs, alcohol, or sex.

# CONNECTING WITH PEERS

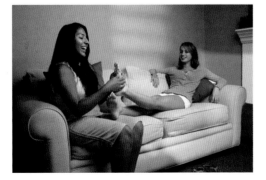

Teenagers enjoy sharing massage with each other as a way to relax, unwind, and connect. They learn to enjoy the many benefits of massage with their friends.

# BODY IMAGE

Bombarded by messages from the media, peers, and even their parents about their bodies and what is beautiful, adolescents can become confused about healthy body image. Home massage takes the focus away from how they look and teaches them the importance of health and wellness. Through the positive touch and unconditional acceptance of the giver, teenagers begin to feel comfortable in their body.

> Following a month of massages, teenagers with bulimia had fewer symptoms of depression, lower anxiety, and lower stress hormones (urinary cortisol levels). Eating habits improved, and they developed improved body image.[26]

# STRESS

Hormonal pressures, parental expectations, peer pressure, and overloaded schedules create stress for teenagers. Although in trying to discover their own identity they seek separation and independence, these children still need the security of their parents' love and acceptance as much as ever. Negotiating this path between adolescence and the independence of adulthood can be extremely stressful for some teenagers. Depression can occur if teenagers don't have the internal and external resources to cope with their feelings. Suicide is the third leading cause of death among teenagers. Home massage can be invaluable for teenagers to reduce stress, lift depression, and relax their mind, body, and spirit.

> Clinical research monitoring brain activity in depressed teenagers revealed that massage therapy had positive effects and indicated that these therapies should be considered in conventional treatment programs for depression.[27, 28]

# IDEAS FOR MASSAGING YOUR TEENAGER

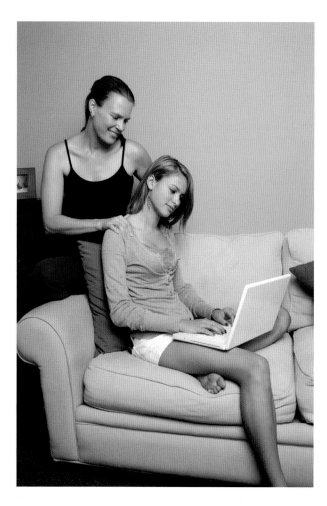

While your teen is bending over the computer doing her homework, gently lay your hands on her shoulders and slowly start massaging her neck and back. This will ease her tense shoulders, increase concentration, and renew her energy.

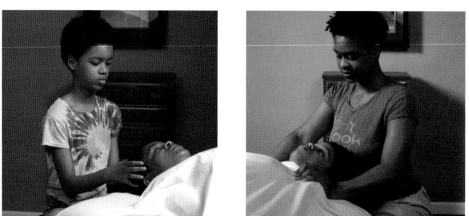

Set aside a time each week to exchange massage with your teenager. She will look forward to this special connection.

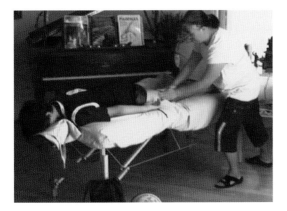

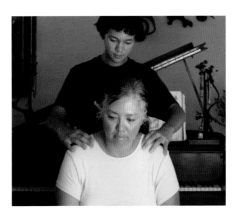

Many teenagers are involved in sports and suffer from tight, over-worked muscles and strains. Invite them to lay on the table or bed, then massage their stressed leg and arm muscles.

Sometimes your teenagers will sur-prise you with a relaxing shoulder massage as a way to let you know they care.

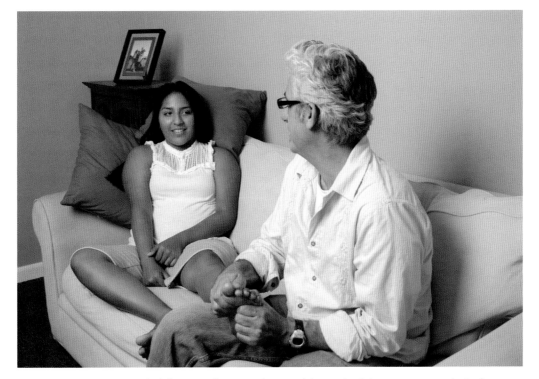

When your teenager is lying on the couch watching television, massage their feet.

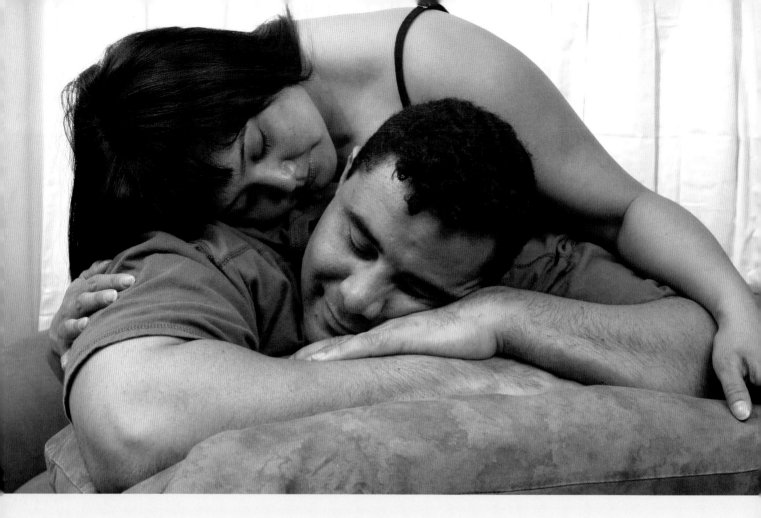

## CHAPTER ELEVEN

# COUPLES

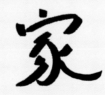

If you don't care for each other,
who will care for you?
—Jack Kornfield

Couples who bring home massage into their lives find that it has renewed their connection with each other and sometimes even saved their relationship. Touch, so important to emotional connection, is sometimes lacking between couples despite living in such close quarters.

Some spouses that have a difficult time communicating with words find they can communicate more easily through the hands-on communication of touch. Home massage between couples inspires closeness and creates mutual relaxation.

# NONSEXUAL TOUCH

Sadly, many couples don't feel comfortable touching except during sex, thus missing out on the healing intimacy of loving touch outside the bedroom. In his definitive book on touch, *Touch Heals*, Ashley Montague writes, "It is sad to reflect that in the western world the only time that many married couples will exhibit nonsexual physical closeness or genuine intimacy is when a serious illness befalls the one or the other." Exercises such as Masters and Johnson's "sensate focus" have been developed to teach couples to lovingly and slowly touch each other everywhere but in the genital and breast areas. These exercises allow couples to give and get sensual stimulation without the burden of performing sexually.

Many relationships fail because couples don't know how to hold each other with this kind of intimate, non-sexual touch. Unfortunately, movies, television, and billboards all suggest that touch equals sex. But even healthy adult sexual touch is based on also receiving the loving, unconditional touch we received as a child from our partner—safe, protective, and nurturing.

Home massage offers couples a way to lovingly connect in a nonthreatening, non-sexual environment. On the massage table, each partner acts from the unwritten agreement that the time together on the table will be non-sexual and non-seducing. This allows each partner to totally relax and enjoy the gift of touch without sexual expectation. No matter how little or how much touch we received as children, we all need a steady diet of this loving touch. Learning how to touch through home massage creates a deeper intimacy and renewed connection between couples.

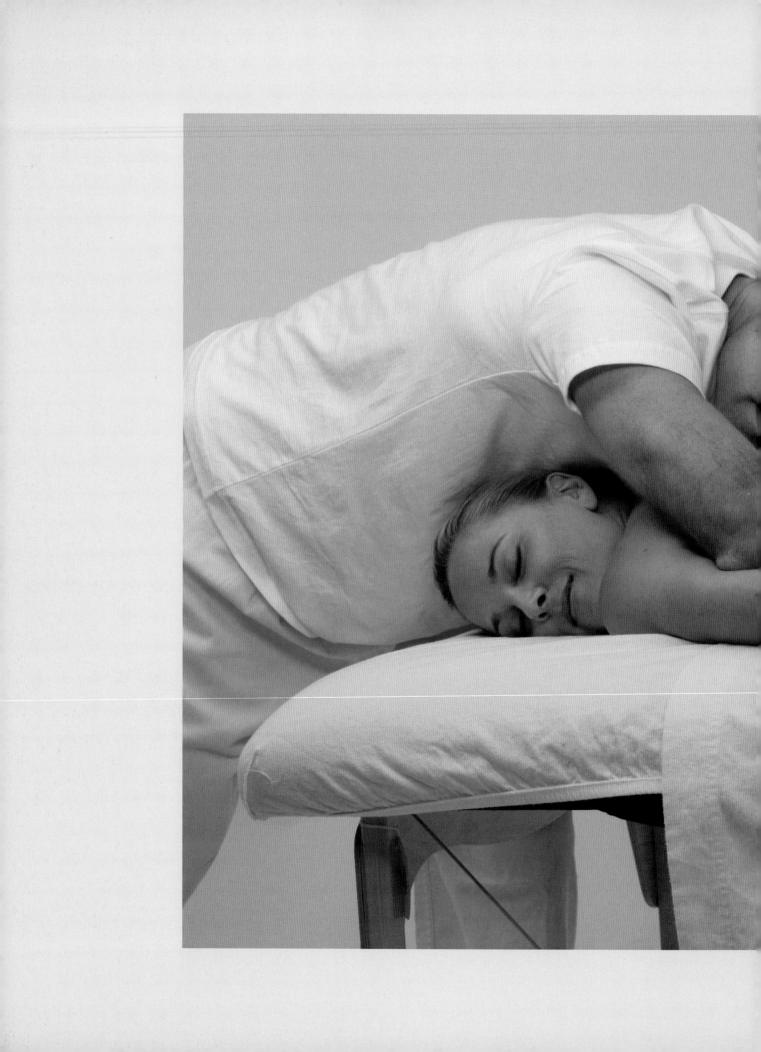

Some couples have learned to communicate with words,
Some have learned to communicate with action,
While others have even learned to communicate with silence.

Yet there are so many
who have never learned
to communicate at all.

—Javan

# IDEAS FOR COUPLES

Many couples find that they are stressed when they return home after a long day at work. Many of them are exhausted and just want to unwind without talking. Giving each other a 10-minute back rub after a long day creates the space to relax and center, offering a positive alternative to silence or withdrawal.

Take the massage table on vacation with you. Exchanging time on the table is even better when you can relax before and after the massage.

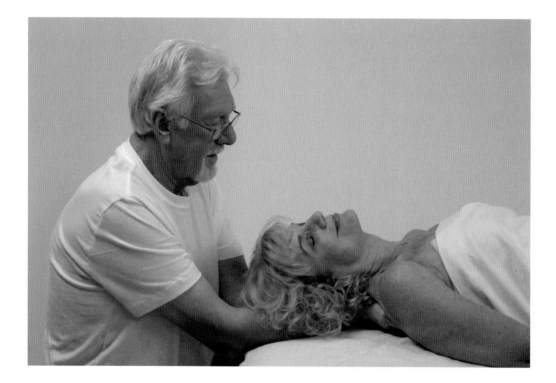

A great gift for a mate for a celebration is a relaxing massage.

Set aside a night each week that is your special time to exchange massage. Use candles, music, and an uncluttered space to set an intimate, relaxing mood. Plan to have time afterwards to completely relax.

Preliminary findings show that couples who massage each other have lower levels of sexual performance anxiety and report increased physical intimacy.[29]

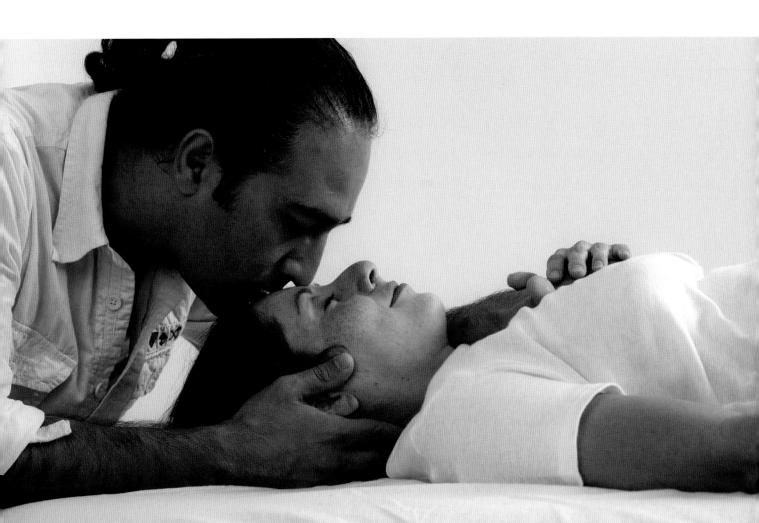

The pressures and responsibilities of family life can wear parents down physically and emotionally. Incorporating massage into the home increases relaxation, renews connection, and soothes the symptoms of stress. With the understood agreement that the massage will be sensual rather than sexual, each person can totally relax into the massage.

New research has found that giving a massage also reduces stress, elevates the mood, and increases your sense of well-being.[30]

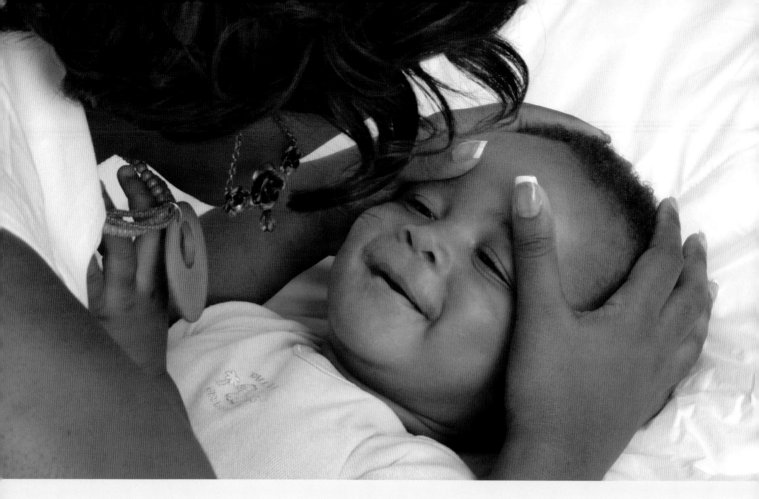

CHAPTER TWELVE

# INFANTS

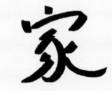

Being touched and caressed,
being massaged,
is food for the infant.
Food as necessary
as minerals, vitamins and proteins.
Deprived of this food,
the name of which is love,
babies would rather die.
And they often do.

—Frederic LeBoyer

For nine months a newborn is in the protected environment of his mother's womb. Birth removes him from this safe environment and delivers him into a strange new world of light, noise, and sudden movements.

Touch lets babies know that they are loved and are safe. Touch is the first developed sense and therefore one of the most highly developed senses in infants. Touching, cuddling, hugging, and stroking are the natural, nurturing ways for parents to bond with their infants. They provide the positive stimulation needed for relaxation and an infant's continuing development. The more a newborn is touched, the better his physical and emotional growth.

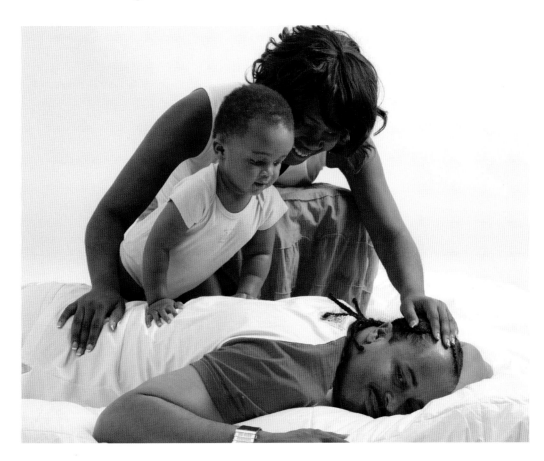

## BENEFITS OF INFANT MASSAGE

Encourages emotional security
Encourages physiological growth
Encourages alertness and responsiveness
Helps infants adapt to their environment
Fosters neurological development
Boosts the immune system
Helps muscle development
Improves motor skills

Promotes social development
Helps prevent colds and infections
Eases agitated babies into sleep
Increases blood flow
Relieves colic and constipation
Calms overstimulated infants
Relieves physical and emotional stress
Promotes a calm disposition

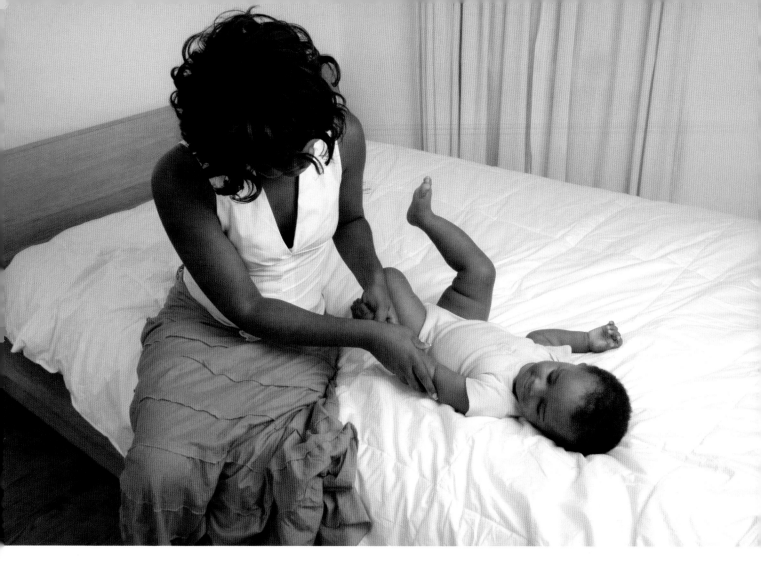

There are no special sequences for massaging a baby. Just adapt your strokes to fit the tiny body. Notice what your baby likes and dislikes. Keep your movements slow and smooth. Do whatever comes naturally. Talk to him lovingly as you massage.

Make sure the room is kept warm and the area well padded. Start with your baby face up so he can see you. Make sure your hands are clean and warm. Remove your jewelry so it doesn't scratch your baby's skin. Use your fingertips or thumbs whenever the area you are working on is too small for your entire hand.

Choose a time when the baby is relaxed to give a massage. The best times are between feedings, after a bath, shortly after waking, right before bedtime, or simply when you both feel the need for closeness. The length of time of the massage depends entirely on how long your baby enjoys the experience. If the baby seems happy, continue. If the baby is fussy, try again later.

Infants who experienced massage therapy spent more time in active alert and active awake states, cried less, and had lower cortisol levels, suggesting lower stress. Over the six-week period, the massage-therapy infants gained more weight, showed greater improvement on emotionality, sociability, and soothability temperament dimensions, and had greater decreases in stress.[31]

# THE HEAD AND FACE

A tender way to begin a massage is with the head and face so you can make eye contact with your baby.

Gently cradle your baby's head in both hands with your thumbs together in the center of the head. Spread your hands to each side.

With the pads of your index fingers, start at the center of the head at the hairline and trace a heart-shape on your baby's face, ending at the chin.

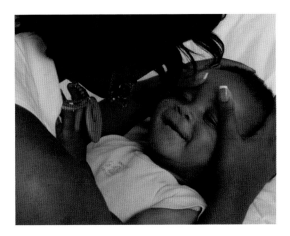

# ARMS AND HANDS

With one hand caress the baby's wrist and gently stroke from the wrist around the shoulders and back down to the wrist. Next, gently squeeze and pull each finger.

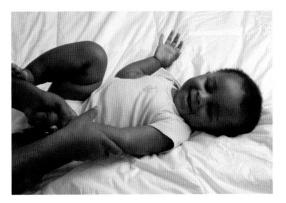

# THE LEGS

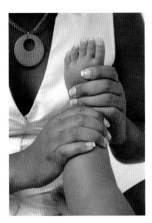

Give your baby's leg a gentle stretch. Caress the baby's foot in your hand. Lower his leg, pushing his knee towards his chest. Then gently extend the leg towards your chest.

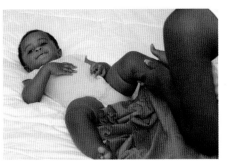

Hold the baby's leg with one hand. With your free hand, start at the ankle and stroke from the ankle to the hip and back down to the ankle.

# TUMMY

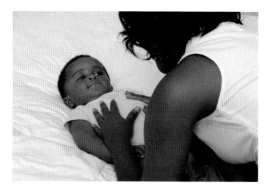

Massaging the belly can expel gas, relieve constipation, and help babies suffering from colic.

Babies digestive systems are quite sensitive. Keep your touch gentle and always clockwise. Massaging counter-clockwise could cause constipation.

# FEET

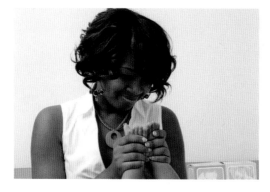

Hold the baby's feet in your hands with your fingers on the top of their feet and your thumbs on the bottom. Use one thumb, following the other thumb to massage from the heel to the toes.

Next, slowly rotate the baby's legs in a bicycle-riding pattern. This can help ease gas pains and has a playful rhythm for both parent and child.

# THE BACK

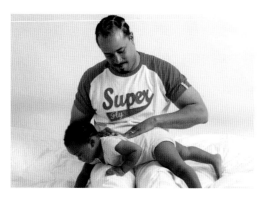

Lie the baby on his stomach across your thighs. With both hands on your baby's back, glide each hand back and forth. Move them in a circular motion and then back and forth in opposite directions.

A pilot study has shown that massage applied to preterm infants with very low birth weights resulted in improved motor skills among those infants who showed especially low motor skills at the start of the study. [32]

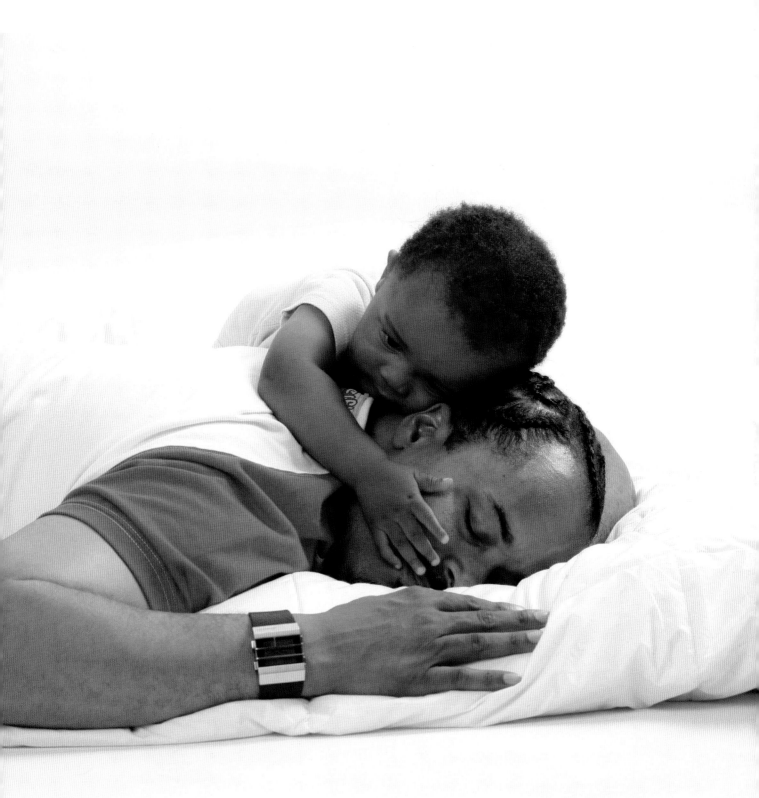

Daddy's turn.

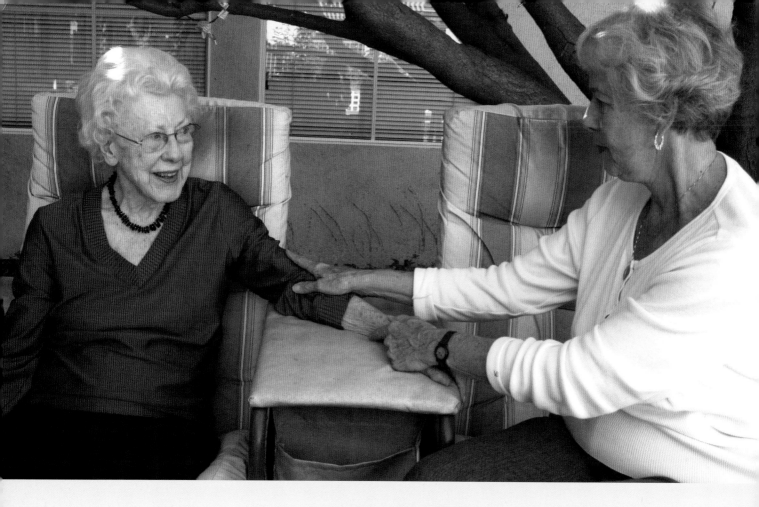

CHAPTER THIRTEEN

# THE ELDERLY

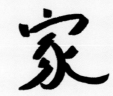

A family with an old person has a living treasure of gold.

—Chinese proverb

Touch is essential for our well-being at all ages, but we receive the least in our later years. Life goes full circle and, just as infants need touch, so do the elderly. Due to the fear of aging in our society, the touch that has nurtured and comforted us earlier in life often dwindles to a token of tenderness or affection.

Massage can greatly enhance the quality of life for the elderly. It can relieve them of depression and loneliness, improve circulation, alleviate stiffness problems, and reduce high blood pressure.

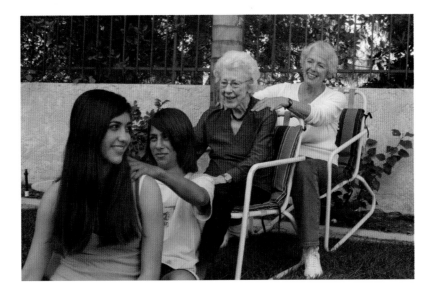

## BENEFITS FOR THE ELDERLY

Stimulates the appetite and digestion
Improves sleep
Reduces joint pain
Relieves swelling caused by fluid retention
Stimulates circulation
Lowers blood pressure
Supports elimination
Improves the skin and relieves dryness and itching
Helps prevent pressure sores
Speeds healing from injuries and surgery
Increases energy
Provides emotional comfort
Increases muscle tone
Eases and deepens breathing
Boosts the immune system

# CARING TOUCH

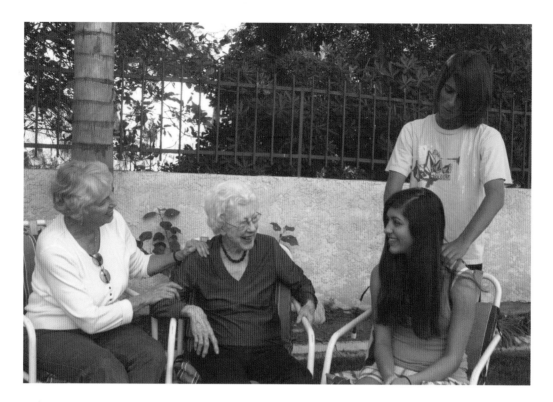

Often just an embrace, light touch, or gentle stroke will make your elderly relative feel loved, appreciated, and nurtured. Caring touch helps the elderly deal with loss, dependency, and a changed body.

The elderly's need to be touched doesn't differ from any other age group. Just remember that an aging body requires extra tender, loving care. If they are bed-ridden or have limited mobility, massage them in their bed or wheelchair. Be soft and gentle—their skin can be fragile and too hard a pressure can tear the skin or cause bruising. Sometimes the skin of the elderly, or that of an ill person, tends to be dryer and often loses some of its absorption capabilities. Often they are taking medications, which can affect absorption as well. Start with very little or no oil. Use light pressure to insure that no harm is done. If massaging on a table, take great care in positioning their body and, once positioned, do not ask them to move. Replace eyewear once you are finished so as not to affect their mobility and balance. Remind them that they could possibly be light-headed after the massage. Suggest that they sit for a while before standing, offering the reason why or assist them to the standing position.

# INCREASING CIRCULATION

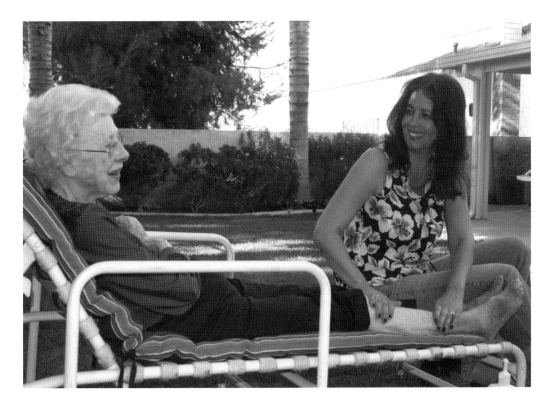

Many elderly relatives or friends may have difficultly walking or don't have full use of their hands due to arthritis. Massaging their feet and hands will increase their circulation. This can be done easily with the person sitting in a chair, on a couch, or in bed. It is best to provide support for the limb that is being massaged. Always begin gently with light pressure and then increase the intensity only if requested. Rotate and flex the wrist or ankle to help improve the mobility of the joints.

Sometimes family members are so excited about being able to help that they forget one of the most important principles: Honor, Repect, and Listen. Before massaging an elderly person, one needs to proceed with a little extra caution. The authors ask that you do no "hands on" until you have read this entire section and the Contraindications on page 78. For further information, refer to our Suggested Reading "for the elderly" section at the end of the book. As always, be sure to check with their doctor if they have any medical conditions or illnesses.

# EASING LONELINESS

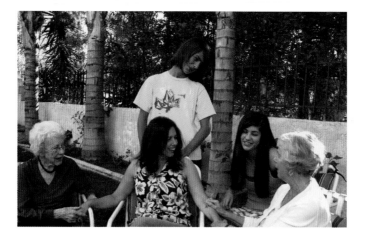

Often there may be no words to make your elderly relative or friend feel better, but a hug, pat on the shoulder, or gentle massage can bring great healing.

Young nursing students tend to avoid touching elderly patients. Our culture associates touch with vibrancy and youth, and so we often don't consider the touch needs of an older person.

A widow after 50 years of marriage might go for weeks and months without being touched. Elderly relatives in a nursing home may feel physically and emotionally isolated from their family. Their spouse may be required to reside in a different room in the facility. Obstacles like wheelchairs and bedside tables may make it difficult to touch our elderly loved ones. Sometimes we may live out of state and are not often able to give the gift of our healing embrace. Or our fast-paced lives are consumed with activity and it seems like we just can't find the time to visit our elderly relatives.

Home massage is a tonic for their body, a comfort to their emotions, and a miracle for their spirits.

> A research study found a correlation between sensory deficits and traits of senility—irritability, memory loss, and careless grooming and eating patterns. Among 42 nursing home residents more than 70 years old, those receiving massages, squeezes, and other affectionate touches were more alert, good-humored, and physically vibrant than those not receiving massage.[33]

# TO GIVE IS TO RECEIVE

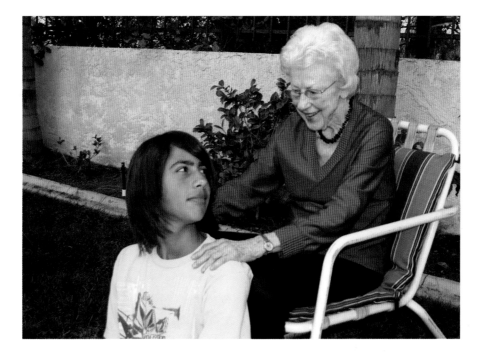

Elderly family members and friends enjoy being the giver of a massage as much as the receiver. In fact, the elderly have been found to actually enjoy giving a massage as much or more because it makes them feel useful.

Research has shown that among hospitalized patients, the psychotic and the elderly were touched the least. The touch they did receive was mostly instrumental to carry out tasks rather than touch to express acceptance, nurturance, and love.[34]

Following a one-month period in which grandparents massaged abused infants, the elderly caregivers experienced increased self-esteem and cortisol levels, improved lifestyle habits, and fewer trips to the doctor's office.[35]

A single 20-minute massage and mobilization protocol focused on the feet and ankles of elderly adults significantly improved their performance on balance tests immediately following touch therapy, according to recent research.[36]

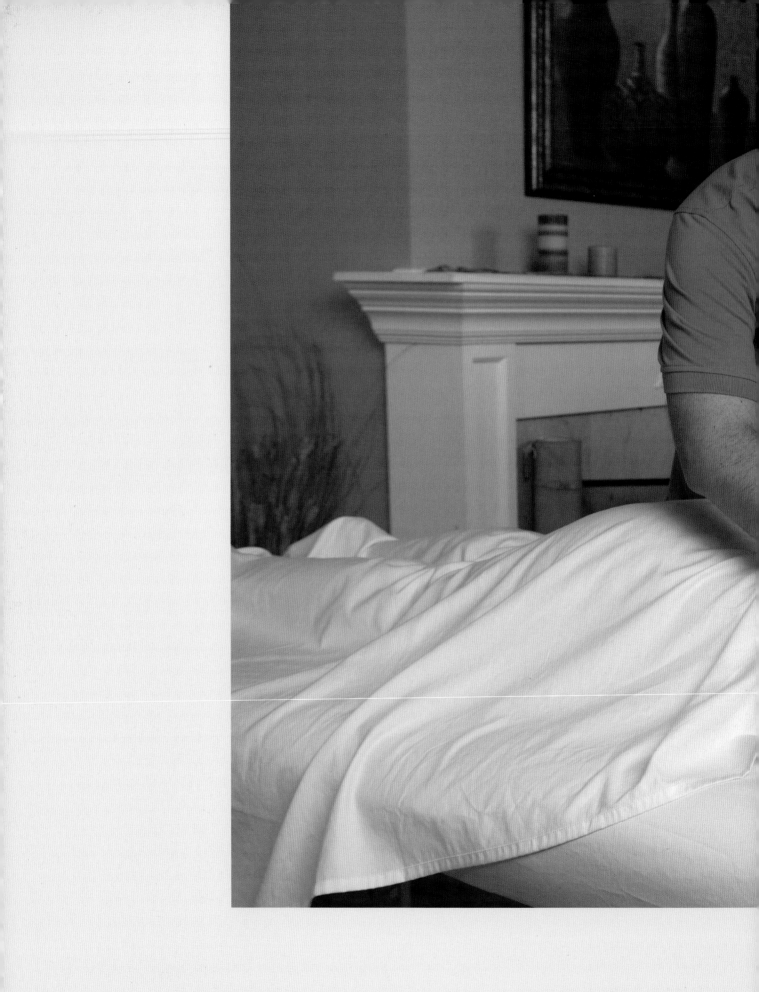

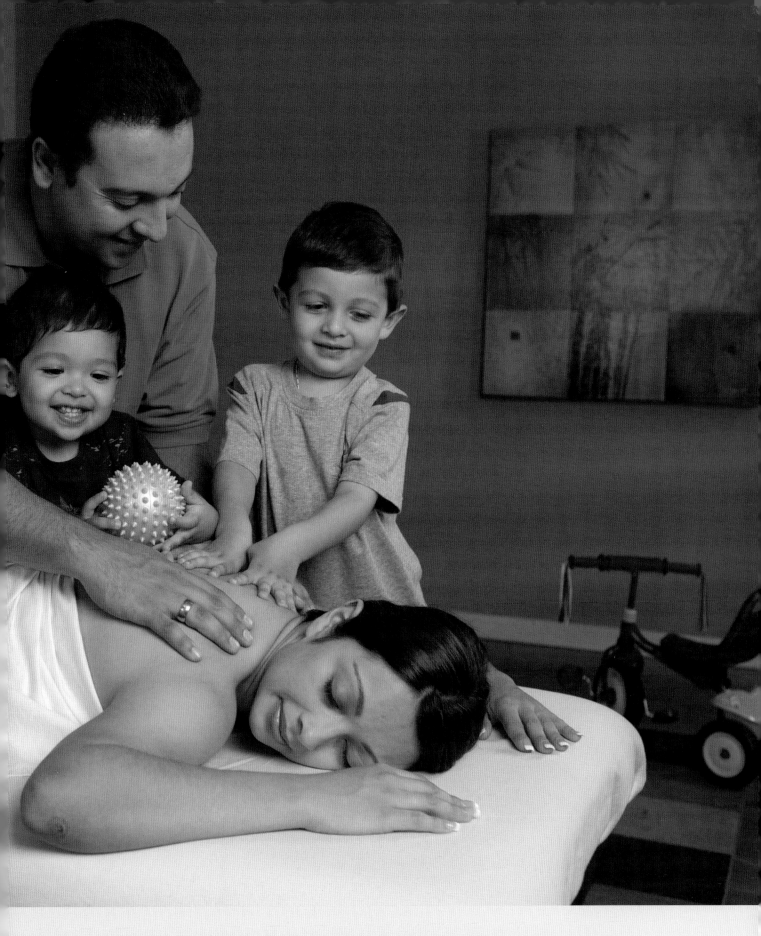

# CONCLUSION

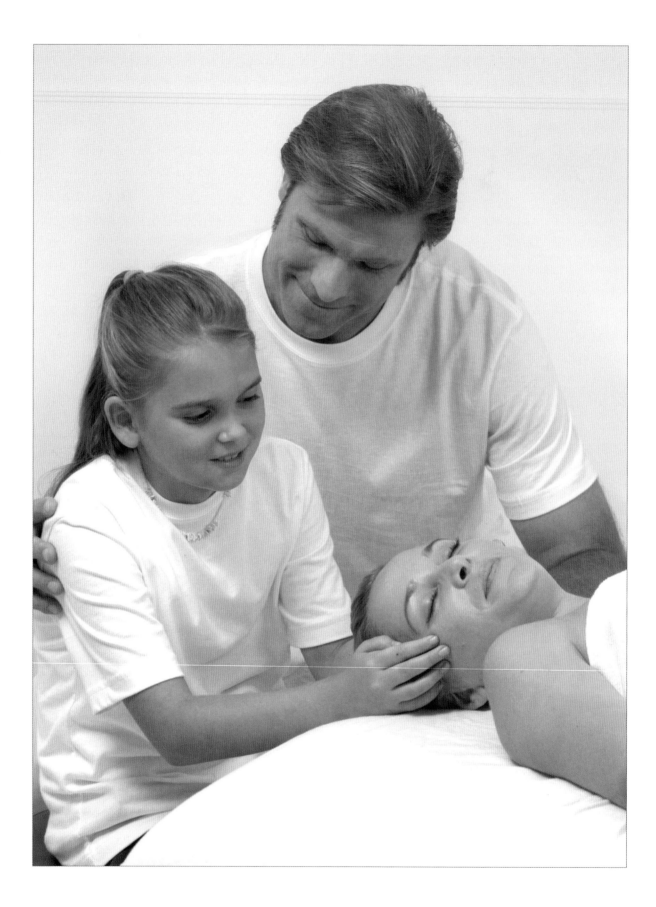

# OUR CHOICE

Man's mind, once stretched by a new idea,
never regains its original dimensions.

*~Oliver Wendell Holmes, Jr.*

There are always many fingers pointing to the same moon. The path to health, connection, and balance has many names but all involve choice.

To close down or open up?

To withdraw or reach out?

To speed up or slow down?

To stay in denial or move into truth?

To isolate or connect?

To live or merely exist?

Touch Communications Home Massage asks us to slow down. It reminds us how relaxation feels. It connects us with those we love. It teaches honor and respect. It returns us to our natural ability to heal ourselves and others through touch.

Thank you for your time.

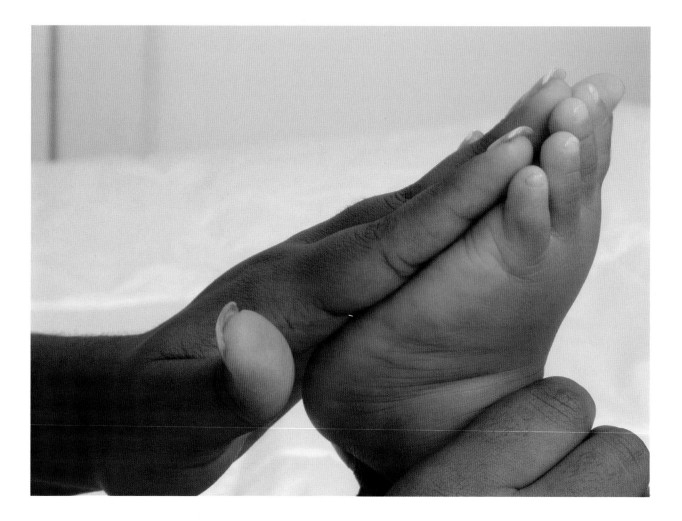

# BIBLIOGRAPHY

Caplan, Mariana, Ph.D. *To Touch Is To Live*. Arizona: Hohm Press, 2002.

Colton, Helen. *The Gift of Touch*. New York: Kensington Press, 1983.

Costa, Larry. *Massage: Mind and Body*. New York: DK Publishing, Inc., 2003.

Davis, Phyllis, Ph.D. *The Power of Touch*. Carlsbad, CA: Hay House, 1999.

Dychtwald, Ken. *Bodymind*. New York: Penguin Putnam Inc., 1950.

Field, Tiffany, Ph.D. *Touch*. Massachusetts: MIT Press, 2003.

Field, Tiffany, Ph.D. *Touch Therapy*. New York: Harcourt Brace, 2000.

Juhan, Deane. *Job's Body: A Handbook for Bodywork*. New York: Station Hill Press, 1987.

Lidell, Lucinda with Sara Thomas, Carola Beresford Cooke, and Anthony Porter. *The Book of Massage*. New York: Simon & Schuster Inc., 1984.

LeBoyer, Frederick. *Loving Hands: The Traditional Art of Baby Massage*. New York: Alfred A. Knopf, 1976.

MacDonald, Gayle. *Medicine Hands: Massage Therapy for People With Cancer*. Scotland: UK. Findhorn Press, 2008.

McIntosh, Nina. *The Educated Heart*. Tennessee: Decatur Bainbridge Press, 1999.

McMahon, James. *The Price of Wisdom*. New York: The Crossroad Publishing Company, 1996.

Montagu, Ashley. *Touching: The Human Significance of the Skin*. New York: Harper and Row Publishers, 1986.

Nelson, Dawn, M.F.A., C.M.T. *From the Heart Through the Hands: The Power of Touch in Caregiving*. Scotland, UK: Findhorn Press, 2009.

Nichols, Michael P Ph.D. *The Lost Art of Listening*. New York: Guilford Press, 1995.

# SUGGESTED READING

## TOUCH AND MASSAGE

Barnard, Kathryn E. and T. Berry Brazelton. *Touch: The Foundation of Experience*. Madison, CT: International Universities Press, 1990.

Caplan, Mariana, PhD. *To Touch Is To Live*. Arizona: Hohm Press, 2002.

Colton, Helen. *The Gift of Touch: How Physical Contact Improves Communication, Pleasure and Health*. New York: Seaview and Putnam, 1983.

Davis, Phyllis K. *The Power of Touch*. Carlbad, CA: Hay House, 1999.

Field, Tiffany M. *Touch in Early Develoment*. Mahwah, NJ: Lawrence Erlbaum Assoc., 1995.

_____, ed. *Touch*. Cambridge, MA: MIT Press, 2001.

_____, ed. *Touch Therapy*. New York: Harcourt Brace, 2000.

Ford, Clyde W. *Compassionate Touch*. New York: Simon and Schuster, 1993.

Finch, Mary Ann. *Care Through Touch: Massage as the Art of Anointing*. New York: Continuum Publishing, 1999.

Heller, Morton, A. *The Psychology of Touch*. Hillsdale, NJ: Lawrence Erlbaum Assoc., 1991.

Josipovici, Gabriel. *Touch*. New Haven, CT: Yale University Press, 1996.

Juhan, Deane. *Job's Body: A Handbook for Bodywork*. Barrytown, NY: Station Hill Press, 1987.

Krieger, Dolores. Ph.D., R.N. *The Therapeutic Touch: How to Use Your Hands to Help or to Heal*. New York: Prentice-Hall, 1979.

Kychinskas, Susan. *The Chemistry of Connection: How the Oxytocin Response Can Help You Find Trust, Intimacy and Love*. Oakland, CA: New Harbinger Publicatoins, Inc., 2009.

Lidell, Lucinda with Sara Thomas, Carola Beresford Booke and Anthony Porter. *The Book of Massage*. New York: Simon & Schuster Inc., 1984.

Montagu, Ashley. *Touching: The Human Significance of the Skin*. New York: Harper and Row Publishers, 1986.

Sayre-Adams, Jean, et al. *The Theory and Practice of Therapeutic Touch*. New York: Churchill Livingstone, 2001.

Simon, Sidney B. *Caring, Feeling, Touching*. Niles, IL: Argues Communications, 1976.

Sullivan, Karin Horgan. *The Healing Power of Touch: The Many Ways Physical Contact Can Cure*. Lincolnwood, Ill: Publications International, Ltd., 1998.

Thomas, Zach. *Healing Touch: The Church's Forgotten Language*. Longville, KY: Westminster John Knox Press, 1994.

Webb, Marcus and Maria. *Healing Touch: A Complete Guide to the Use of Touch Therapies that Promote Well-Being*. New York: Sterling Publishing Company, 1999.

## INFANT MASSAGE

Ady, Mary. *An Infant Massage Guidebook: For Well, Premature, and Special Needs Babies.* Bloomington, IN: Authorhouse, 2008.

Heath, Alan and Nicki Bainbridge. *Baby Massage: The Calming Power of Touch.* London, England: DK Adult, 2004.

Heller, Sharon, Ph.D. *The Vital Touch: How Intimate Contact With Your Baby Leads To Happier, Healthier Development.* Henry Holt and Co. LLC, 1997.

LeBoyer, Frederick. *Loving Hands. The Traditional Art of Baby Massage.* New York: Alfred A. Knopf, 1976.

Mc Clure, Vimala Schneider. *Infant Massage: A Handbook for Loving Parents.* Bantam, 2000.

Reese, Suzanne and Milne. *Baby Massage: Soothing Strokes for Healthy Growth.* New York, NY: Viking Press, 2006.

Staerker, Paul. *Tender Touch: Massage Your Baby to Health and Happiness.* Singapore: Twickenham Media Masters, 1999.

Toporek, Robert. *New Book of Baby and Child Massage.* Philadelphia, PA: Running Press, 2001.

## PET MASSAGE

Ayrault, Megan, LMP. *The Dog Lovers Guide to Massage: What Your Dog Wants You to Know.* Kirkland, WA: All About Animal Massage, 2009.

Hourdebaigt, Jean-Pierre. *Canine Massage: A Complete Reference Manual.* Wenatchee, WA: Direct Book Service, 2003.

Prasad, Kathleen and Fulton, Elizabeth. *Animal Reiki: Using Energy to Heal the Animal in Your Life.* Berkeley Press: Ulysses Press, 2006.

Robertson, Julia. *Physical Therapy and Massage for the Dog.* New York, NY: Thieme/Manson, 2011.

## STRESS

Forman, Jeffrey W. *Managing Physical Stress with Therapeutic Massage.* Clifton Park, NY: Milady, 2006.

Kavanagh, Wendy. *Massage Basics: How to Treat Aches and Pains, Stress and Flagging Energy.* London, England: Hamlyn, Revised Edition, 2009.

Inkeles: Gordon. *Unwinding: Super Massage For Stress Control.* New York: Grove PR, 1998.

Roseberry, Monica. *Massage: Simple Solutions for Everyday Stresses.* London: Aurum Press Ltd., 2005.

# PREGNANCY

Osbourne, Carole. *Pregnancy: Pre and Perinatal Massage Therapy.* Wolter Kluwer, Philadelphia, PA: Lippincott, Williams & Wilkins, 2009.

Stillerman, Elaine. *A Handbook for Relieving the Discomforts of Pregnancy.* Brooklyn, New York: Delta, 1992.

Waters, Bette. *Massage During Pregnancy.* St. Augustine, Florida: Bluewaters Press, 2009.

# COUPLES

Horan, Peggy Morrison. *Connecting Through Touch: The Couples Massage Book.* Oakland, CA: New Harbinger, 2007.

# CHILDREN

Carlson, Frances M. National Association For The Education of Young Children. *Essential Touch: Meeting the Needs of Young Children.* Washington, DC: National Association for the Education of Young Children.

Chapman, Gary. *The Five Love Languages of Teenagers.* Chicago, Illinois: Northfield Publishing, 2000

Martin, Chia. *The Art of Touch: A Masage Manual for Young People.* Prescott, AZ: Holm Press, 1996.

# CAREGIVING, ILLNESS, THE ELDERLY

Babcock, Elise NeeDell. *When Life Becomes Precious: A Guide for Loved Ones and Friends of Cancer Patients.* New York, NY: Bantam Books, 1997.

Catlin, Ann, LMT, OTR. *Sensitive Massage: Reclaiming the Human Touch in Caregiving.* Compassionate Touch, Springfield, MO 2010. DVD

MacDonald Gayle, M.S,, L.M.T. *Medicine Hands: Massage Therapy for People with Cancer.* Findhorn, Scotland: Findhorn Press, Revised Second Edition, 2006.

Meisler, Deitrich and Meiia, Else. *Massaging the Alzheimer's Patient.* Daybreak Geriatric Massage Institute. DVD.

Nelson, Dawn, M.F.A., C.M.T. *From the Heart Through the Hands: The Power of Touch in Caregiving.* Findhorn, Scotland: Findhorn Press, Third Edition, 2009.

Rose, Mary Kathleen. *Comfort Touch: Massage for the Eldery and Ill.* Lippincott, Williams and Wilkins, 2006.

Thompson, M. Keith, M.D. *Caring For An Elderly Relative: A Guide to Home Care.* New York: Prentice-Hall, 1986.

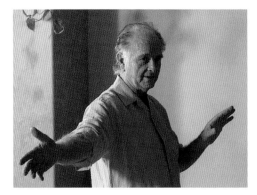

Co-founder of TCHM, Chuck was a nationally certified massage therapist with a private practice in Long Beach, California. He was an instructor at the University of Irvine and the Shiatsu Massage School of California. Chuck taught and lived from the heart. His message was reverence, honor, respect, acceptance and love. Although he has gone on to his next jouney, his vision continues with family members, friends and his numerous students. The ripples from his "stone" still flow outwards, touching and transforming many more lives.

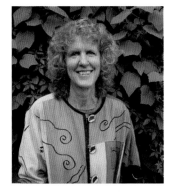

Suzette Hodnett, M.S. co-founder of TCHM, has a background as a licensed psychotherapist, professional artist and Tai Chi Sandan instructor. She currently works as a Life Coach, blending her experience to bring emotional and physical health to youth and adults. With Jackie Sloan, CMT, she offers retreats, lectures and workshops nationwide to promote relaxation, connection, and the healing power of touch.

If you would like to get in touch with Suzette and share your thoughts about this book and about your experience with massage and touch:

Email: suz4tchm@aol.com

Website: www.tchomemassage.com

Please contact us if you would like to schedule a massage workshop, lecture, retreat, or to order additional home massage products such as:

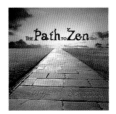

*The Path to Zen: Songs of Serenity (CD)*
by Sonic Zion

Enjoy this relaxing music while you exchange massage and relax throughout the day.

# REFERENCES

[1] Suomi SJ, Brown CC et al. "The role of touch in rhesus monkey social development." In *The Many Facets of Touch*, Johnson & Johnson Pediatric Roundtable. 1984:10:41-56.

[2] Schanberg S, and Field T. "Maternal deprivation and supplemental stimulation." In *Stress and Coping Across Development*, Field T, McCabe P, and Schneiderman N, eds. Hillsdale, NJ: Erlbaum; 1988.

[3] Suomi SJ. "Genetic and maternal contributions to individual differences in rhesus monkey biobehavioral development." In *Perinatal Development: A Psychobiological Perspective*, Krasnegor N et al., eds. New York: Academic Press; 1987:397-420.

[4] Fairbanks LA. "Early experience and cross-generational continuity of mother-infant contact in vervet monkeys." *Developmental Psychobiology.* 1989:27:669-681.

[5] Prescott, J. W. (1990). "Affectional bonding for the prevention of violent behaviors: Neurobiological, psychological and religious/spiritual determinants." In L. J. Herzberg, G. F. Ostrum, & J. Roberts Field (Eds.), *Violent behavior: Assessment and intervention (Vol. 1).* Great Neck, NY: PMA Publishing Co.

[6] Hernandez-Reif, M., Ironson, G., Field, T., Katz, G., Diego, M., Weiss, S., Fletcher, M., Schanberg, S. & Kuhn, C. (2003). "Breast cancer patients have improved immune functions following massage therapy." *Journal of Psychosomatic Research,* 57, 45-52.

[7] Ironson, G., Field, T., Scafidi, F., Hashimoto, M., Kumar, M., Kumar, A., Price, A., Goncalves, A., Burman, I., Tetenman, C., Patarca, R., & Fletcher, M. A. (1996). "Massage therapy is associated with enhancement of the immune system's cytotoxic capacity." *International Journal of Neuroscience,* 84, 205-217.

[8] Diego, M.A., Field, T., Hernandez-Reif, M., Hart, S., Brucker, B., Field, Tory, Burman, I. (2002). "Spinal cord patients benefit from massage therapy." *International Journal of Neuroscience,* 112, 133-142.

[9] Uppsala University Department of Public Health and Caring Sciences, in Uppsala, Sweden. Authors: Dan Hasson, Bengt Arentz, Lena Jelveus and Bo Edelstam. Originally published in *Psychotherapy and Psychosomatics,* 2004, Vol. 73, pp. 17-24.

[10] Hernandez,-Reif, M., Field, T., Krasnegor, J., Theakston, H., and Burman, I. (2000) "Chronic lower back pain is reduced and range of motion increased after massage therapy." *International Journal of Neuroscience* 99: 1-15.

[11] Pilot study, Cedars Sinai Hospital Medical Center, Los Angeles.

[12] Hernandez-Reif, M., Field, T., Krasnegor, J. & Theakston, H. (2000). "High blood pressure and associated symptoms were reduced by massage therapy." *Journal of Bodywork and Movement Therapies,* 4, 31-38.

[13] Field, T.M., Hernandez-Reif, M., Hart, S., Theakston, H., Schanberg, S., Kuhn, C, and Burman, I. (1999) "Pregnant woman benefit from massage therapy." *Journal of Psychosomatic Obstetrics and Gynecology,* 20: 31-28.

[14] University of Colorado, National Institutes of Health and National Center for Complementary and Alternative Medicine. Originally published in the *Annals of Internal Medicine* 2008:149: 369-379.

[15] Health Sciences School, Universidad Granada, Spain; Universidad Rey Juan Carlos, Alcorcón, Madrid, Spain; Franklin Pierce University, Concord, New Hampshire; Concord Hospital, New Hampshire; Regis University, Denver, Colorado; University Hospital San Cecilio, Granada, Spain. Originally published in *Journal of Manipulative and Physiological Therapeutics,* September 2009:32 (7): 527-535.

[16] Dr. Cronfalk, Karolinska Institute. "Hand and foot massages consoled bereaved relatives." *Journal of Clinical Nursing,* April 4, 2010.

[17] *The Pet Arthritis Chronicle.* Volume One. Issue 7.

[18] Dr. von Haunersches Kinderspital Department of Pediatric Neurology and Developmental Medicine; Friedrich-Baur-Institute Department of Neurology; Institute for Medical Informatics, Biometrics and Epidemiology; and Ludwig-Maximilians-University, Munich, Germany. Originally published in the *Journal of Child Neurology* (April 2009) 24(4): 406-409.

[19] Field, T.M., Lasko, D., Mundy, P., Henteleff, T., Talpins, s., and Dowling, M. (1996) "Autistic children's atentiveness and responsivity improved after touch therapy." *Journal of Autism and Developmental Disorders* 27 (3): 333-338.

[20] Escalna, A., Field, T.M., Singer-Strunk, R., Cullen, C., and Hartshorn, K. (2001) "Autism symptoms decrease following massage therapy." *Journal of Autism and Developmental Disability.*

[21] Field, T.M., Shaw, K.H., and La Greca, A. (1996) "Massage therapy lowers blood glucose levels in children with diabetes mellitus." *Diabetes spectrum* 10: 237-239.

[22] Field, T.M., Henteleff, T., Hernandez-Reif, M., Martinez, E., Mavunda, K., Kuhn, C., and Schanberg, S. (1998) "Children with asthma have improved pulmonary functions after massage therapy." *Journal of Pediatrics* 132: 854-858.

[23] University of Arizona, Tucson, College of Medicine; Cancer Center, Shands Hospital at the University of Florida, Gainesville. Originally published in the *International Journal of Therapeutic Massage and Bodywork* June 2009 2(2): 7-14.

[24] Hart, S.; Field, T.; Hernandez-Reif, M.; & Lundy, B. (1998). "Preschoolers' cognitive performance improves following massage." *Early Child Development and Care,* 143, 59-64.

[25] Field, T.M., Quintino, O., Hernandez-Reif, M., and Koslovsky, G. (1998). "Adolescents with attention deficit hyperactivity disorder benefit from massage therapy." *Adolescence* 33: 103-10

[26] Field, T.M., Schanberg, S., Kuhn, C., Fierro, K., Henteleff, T., Mueller, C., Yando, R., Shaw, S., and Burman, I. (1998). "Bulimic adolescents benefit from massage therapy." *Adolescence* 33: 555:-563.

[27] Department of Neuroscience, Uppsala University, Sweden; Axelson's Gymnasics Institute, Stockholm, Sweden; Department of Animal Health and Welfare, University of Agriculture, Skara, Sweden. Originally published in *Acta Paediatrica* (2008) 97, 1265-1269.

[28] Field, T.M., Morrow, C., Valdeon, C., Larson, S., Kuhn, C., and Schanberg, S. (1992). "Massage therapy reduces anxiety in child and adolescent psychiatric patients." *Journal of the American Academy of Child and Adolescent Psychiatry* 31: 125-131.

[29] Kleinman, Susan. *The Pleasure—and the Power—of Human Touch.* Based on research at TRI, University of Miami School of Medicine.

[30] Shaw, Allison. *Couples Massages.* Based on research at TRI, University of Miami School of Medicine.

[31] Field, T., Grizzle, N., Scafidi, F. Abrams, S., Richardson, S., Kuhn, C., & Schanberg, S. (1996). "Massage therapy for infants of depressed mothers." *Infant Behavior and Development,* 19, 107-112.

[32] Physiotherapy and pediatric departments, Princess Margaret Hospital, Hong Kong; and Department of Rehabilitation Sciences, Hong Kong Polytechnic University, Hong Kong. Originally published in *Pediatrics International* (Sept. 15, 2009).

[33] O'Neil, P.M., and Calhoun, K.S. (1975). "Sensory deficits and behavioral deterioration in senescence." *Journal of Abnormal Psychology* 84: 579-82.

[34] Barnette K. "The effects of touch as they relate to nursing." *Nursing Research* 1972; 21:102-110.

[35] Field, T.M., Hernandez-Reif, M., Quintino, O., Schanberg, S., and Kuhn, C. (1998). "Elder retired volunteers benefits from giving massage therapy to infants." *Journal of Applied Gerontology* 17: 229-239.

[36] Laboratoire Santé Plasticité Motricité, Université Joseph Fourier-Grenoble, Grenoble, France; Ecole de Kinésthérapie du Centre Hospitalier Universitaire de Grenoble, Grenoble, France; Hôpital de Saint-Laurent-du-Pont, Saint-Laurent-du-Pont, France; Service de Rhumatologie du Centre Hospitalier Universitaire de Genéve, Genéve, Switzerland; Service de Rhumatologie du Centre Hospitalier Universitaire de Grenoble, Grenoble, France. Originally published in *Manual Therapy* (2009).

# ACKNOWLEDGMENTS

Our TC Home Massage co-founder, Jackie Sloan, who continually inspires others to discover that touch is their own innate magic. If it were not for Jackie there would be no TCHM. Jackie is responsible for bringing a sense of community, connection, and relationship to our workshops. She keeps the message of home massage alive. Though not an author of this book, she was always there for support and played a critical role in the development and editing of the massage techniques.

Jim Chenevey, CEO and Tomas Nani, Founder of Earthlite, Inc., for their support of home massage and vision of "healing humanity through touch."

Our photographer, Tim Neighbors, for his dedication, attention to detail, and commitment to high standards.

The enthusiastic support of our one-woman fan club, Lourdes Flamino, and her uncanny ability to bring the right people together at the right time.

Dr. Jack Ebner for the use of his wonderful yoga studio to hold our workshops and to Nancy Isabel for her warm smile and constant "behind the scenes" assistance.

To Findhorn Press, our talented friends "across the pond," who launched our dream to reality.

Liza Macawili, makeup artist (cover and inserts), for her high standards and keen eye.

The forerunners on the subject of touch—Ashley Montague, Tiffany Field and Mariana Caplan—who helped shape our vision to bring massage into the home.

Those of you who have taken the time to read this book and begin your touch journey.

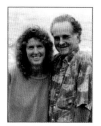

Our heartfelt appreciation,
—Chuck Fata and Suzette Hodnett

My loving thanks to...

My co-author, Suzette Hodnett, whose hard work, creativity, calm, sensitivity, vision, and unique talents, continue to take TCHM to greater depths.

Dr. Vincent Medici for sharing his wealth of knowledge of the art of healing with me and for bringing me back to health.

My children, who inspired me to continue my vision to have massage become an integral part of family life.

My students, who continue to show me the limitless possibilities of rediscovering touch through the principles of Touch Communications Home Massage.

—Chuck Fata

---

A special thank you to those who have touched my life...

My co-author, best friend, travelling companion, and partner who showed me what it feels like to love and be loved. Thank you for your healing heart and hands. I miss you.

My parents, three sisters (Cricket, Jeannine, and Kerry), and nieces and nephews (Tally, Kerrigan, Molly, and Brian) whose willingness to "take turns" continually allowed family touch through massage to be a part of my childhood and adult life. And for my fond memories of the "octopus"—four people and eight hands melting me into relaxed bliss.

My deep appreciation to my Tai Chi teacher, Sensei Frank Mc Gouirk, of the Aikido-ai Institute in Whittier, for his many years of nurturing support, light-hearted humor, excellent teaching about presence and connection, and insight into the many layers of this art.

All my clients, students and friends who continually remind me of the importance of loving touch in our lives.

—Suzette Hodnett

# INDEX

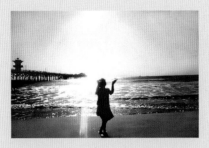

Touch is as essential to us as sunlight.

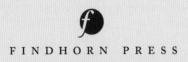

FINDHORN PRESS

*Life-Changing Books*

www.findhornpress.com